# Craniosacral Therapy
## for Babies and Small Children

# Craniosacral Therapy
## *for* Babies *and*
## Small Children

ETIENNE AND NEETO PEIRSMAN

FOREWORD BY

John E. Upledger, DO, OMM

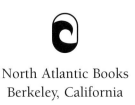

North Atlantic Books
Berkeley, California

Published by
North Atlantic Books
P.O. Box 1232
Berkeley, California 94712

Translated from the Dutch by the authors
Photos by Neeto Peirsman
Cover and book design © Ayelet Maida, A/M Studios
Drawings on pages 7–10, 46, 48, 51, 54, and 55 by Dominique Degrangés, from *Craniosacral Biodynamics,* vol.2, by Franklyn Sills. Reproduced by permission of North Atlantic Books.
Drawing on page 13 by Marie-Andree Brands
Printed in Singapore
Distributed to the book trade by Publishers Group West

*Craniosacral Therapy for Babies and Small Children* is sponsored by the Society for the Study of Native Arts and Sciences, a nonprofit educational corporation whose goals are to develop an educational and crosscultural perspective linking various scientific, social, and artistic fields; to nurture a holistic view of arts, sciences, humanities, and healing; and to publish and distribute literature on the relationship of mind, body, and nature.

North Atlantic Books' publications are available through most bookstores. For further information, call 800-337-2665 or visit our website at www.northatlanticbooks.com.

Substantial discounts on bulk quantities are available to corporations, professional associations, and other organizations. For details and discount information, contact our special sales department.

*Library of Congress Cataloging-in-Publication Data*
Peirsman, Etienne.
[Cranio-sacraaltherapie voor baby's en kinderen. English]
Craniosacral therapy for babies and small children / by Etienne and Neeto Peirsman ; foreword by John E. Upledger.
p. ; cm.
Includes bibliographical references.
ISBN-13: 978-1-55643-597-3 (pbk.)   ISBN-10: 1-55643-597-5 (pbk.)
1. Craniosacral therapy. 2. Infants—Diseases—Chiropractic treatment. 3. Children—Diseases—Chiropractic treatment.   I. Peirsman, Neeto. II. Title.
[DNLM: 1. Manipulation, Osteopathic—methods. 2. Cerebrospinal Fluid. 3. Child. 4. Infant. 5. Sacrum. 6. Skull.   WB 940 P379c 2006a]
RZ399.C73P45 2006
615.8'2--dc22                                          2006011309

2 3 4 5 6 7 8 9 TWP 12 11 10 09 08 07

*Alles van waarde is weerloos.*
– Lucebert

*All beings are from the very beginning Buddhas.*
– Hakuin

*Remember, when you are speaking to a baby,*
*you are speaking to a soul and not to an idiot.*
– Anubhava

# Contents

# Foreword

*Craniosacral Therapy for Babies and Small Children* is a wonderful book about human as well as other mammalian reproduction observations. Together, the authors have developed an excellent body of knowledge in the area of care for both mothers and babies. Their methods and knowledge are based in part on scientific facts, in part on their own discoveries. They have developed many of their supportive methods and treatments as they observed problems that arise during the birth process. They then allowed their creative and intuitive abilities to develop what is now the subject matter of an excellent treatise on what a skilled hands-on therapist can do to ensure that babies have the optimum structural space in which to develop.

This book goes from the physical and physiological to the spiritual aspects of the stages of life, most of which are more closely related to conception, pregnancy, delivery, and post-partum health. Illustrated with excellent action photographs, this book is well worth a read as well as a view.

Enjoy.

– John E. Upledger, DO, OMM
Palm Beach Gardens, Florida

# Preface

It took me more than six years before I, as a CranioSacral (CS) therapist, dared to look at babies, let alone touch them. Babies cry . . . that is not for me, I decided. I have known this uneasiness my whole life. A baby who screams has always had a paralyzing effect on me.

Babies were always too real and expected a real way of interaction. Making funny faces and doing baby talk was not the way that I wanted to interact with them, and I didn't know another way, so I decided to stay out of their way.

After I had worked for years as a CS therapist, slowly mothers with babies started to come to me. Luckily for me I had a wife at my side who took me by the hand and showed me how to deal with these creatures. Again and again she told me, "You really have to listen to them, and welcome them. Talk to them softly while you look at them. And especially, don't talk to the mother at the same time." I have seen her hold a baby close to her heart and tell it, "Welcome to this life, I'm so glad you are here."

A baby is just as conscious as you and I, only it is imprisoned in a body that has very limited communication possibilities. When I felt comfortable in myself and could look beyond the little body of the baby, I saw a soul that had just started its journey in this world. I also started to see that this soul came here with eyes that told about silence and space and pure love. It is those eyes that literally light up if you look inside. That clarity, that wakefulness, that innocence is always present. Keeping that clarity is what education should be about.

Neeto, my wife, says this: "All babies are from the very beginning perfect." This original perfection is not always evident with some babies after birth. And it's about this—finding back space and possibilities, giving back and finding back of the original potential—that is what this book is about. I therefore want to thank Neeto, because she taught me not to be afraid of communicating with these wonderful prophets of love and intelligence.

This is not a scientific document. This is a step-by-step guide to the craniosacral treatment of babies and the birth of love. You will also find in these pages our own working philosophy, which is based on our experience of meditation and common sense.

Some people may feel that certain explanations are oversimplified and elementary; I do speak about many things as though I am talking to a five-year-old. This is because some very fundamental and elementary precepts are missing from our understanding of mothering and the birth process, completely overlooked and overridden by the medical-pharmaceutical establishment and other relevant professionals who have hijacked the natural animal instinct and common sense about birth: the flurry of activity around the ordinary birth scene, picking up the newborn by the feet and putting it unceremoniously on a cold metal scale to weigh it, quickly drying off the wetness with harsh scrubs, putting a cap on its head, pricking its foot, and putting drops in its eyes, etc., all with the supercilious officiousness of the consummate professional! How could it not be challenged? Have mothers gone to sleep?

– Etienne Peirsman

# Acknowledgments

My sincere thanks go to Emy ten Seldam from the Ankh Hermes Publishing house in the Netherlands for first asking me to write a book on CS therapy. I never liked writing, but I came to love it.

My teachers in the Cranial field were Badhrena Tschumi, who really immersed me, and Dr. John Upledger, who took me in and is still my teacher. Thank you both for setting me on my way. I'd also like to thank all the people at North Atlantic Books for making the work of Love and Hope available for all to see, especially Sarah Serafimidis, Yvonne Cárdenas, and Kathy Glass.

Everything I know about babies I learned from my companion, Neeto. She taught me how to communicate with them and above all, she gave me the confidence to do this work and to keep on developing my skills.

Also I'd like to thank all the people who stood in my way and forced me towards freedom. You are many and I am grateful for the challenge.

Finally, I thank all those newborns and small children who have come to us: to Neeto and me. You have been our Zen Masters.

They come to be greeted, they come to be treated.

They come to remember, and through them, we also remember!

– Etienne Peirsman

I would like to give special thanks to Dr. Bob and Mrs. Ruth Ross, who guided me into discovering the quality and depth that babies possess upon entering this world. Many years ago I was very lucky to work as an assistant with them in the Upstate Medical Center in Syracuse, New York. Together they had created and administered a unique residential treatment program for blind children. It was there that I learned the importance of respect, trust and contact with children. Their patience and skill with babies and children was taken as a gift to me throughout my own motherhood and subsequent work with children. These were extremely important lessons about life and how to value it.

These prior experiences also enabled me to see the perfect use of these lessons in CS therapy. My photos were taken with the intention of highlighting this trust and contact between therapist and child.

– Neeto Peirsman

# Introduction

I just saw on TV a class of six-year-olds that had a visit from two policemen on their horses. All the kids were looking in pure wonder at these enormous animals. What happens to us when we grow up? It looks as if we all take a big detour, via neuroses, to reach that innocence again, with a bit of luck.

This book is about the birth of love between mother and child, and about the basic possibilities of love in our world. But ... how do you make sure that love can appear? And what do you do if your baby is inconsolable from the very beginning and you feel yourself to be without any power and finally totally without strength?

What goes beyond the tricks of therapy? What therapy is, is the respect for the being that is being touched. This respect gives the baby (and all onlookers) the feeling of "I am being seen; I am recognized as the soul that I am." And this makes it easier for him or her to accept this strange and threatening world.

We automatically give our children this security if we give mother and child a chance to connect with each other at birth. If the mammalian brain is activated at birth then there is no reason for stress, and at that moment love, chemically induced via hormones, gets installed on their "hard drives."

When I started working for the first time with the CS system and its rhythms, a world of wonderment opened up for me. The CS system is the oldest, deepest and most primitive system in the body. Shortly after conception when the cells start to build the body, the nervous system (within it the CS system) is the first thing that forms. Out of this, building blocks appear that will form the whole body.

When a newborn child passes through the birth canal, it is compressed completely. Sometimes little bones end up at the wrong spot or slide over each other and stay stuck. Of course this hinders the brain because there is not enough space to grow. Compression can also happen to the spinal column or at both places simultaneously. Our therapy looks for and finds these stuck places and we release them. By putting our hands on the baby and connecting with its CS system we give an enormous boost of energy to the circle that connects us to the baby. This creates a clarity that will take the treatment to its point.

What became very clear to me was that this therapy was so easy to learn. Curiosity was enough to start with, and I soon found that the simplicity and clarity was such a big attraction for the body, it was also irresistible for me. I wanted to be in that clarity and simpleness. It is mindlessness itself, the meditative state, which differentiates my work from most osteopathic approaches.

Up to now we have educated hundreds of therapists who practice from out of their own knowledge and experience. Because they went through their own problems, they are able to guide every client out of almost every problem that arises. We give advice and treat mother and baby before and after birth.

**It is absolutely not wise for these techniques to be used or tried out by anybody who just reads this book. All techniques described in this book are meant for CS therapists.**

Our experience taught us, though, that anybody who is really interested can learn to apply these techniques safely. Education and practice are absolutely required. All techniques which we learn in CS therapy, including reliving our own birth, are part of the education of the CS therapist. By doing this we can avoid the possibility of the unsolved birth traumas of the therapist playing an unconscious part in the treatments.

Finally, it is our goal to train as many people as possible in these natural and simple techniques in order to bring back the "wise women" that have been exterminated by the churches and supplanted by the medical profession, and give them back their rightful place in our society.

—Etienne Peirsman

Every baby that comes for a session is a unique new human being. This small body does not have the communication skills that we have. And this is sometimes enormously frustrating for both parties. Communication with the mother happens mostly via smells, touch and sounds that will guarantee trust and security. As I look deep into the baby's eyes, I start to make slow sounds. I welcome the baby and this doesn't necessarily need to be with words; it is looking and letting my energy flow, touching through my eyes.

During the whole session I try to be connected totally with the baby through the spinal cord, eyes and sound. When I

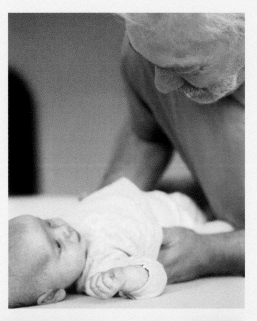

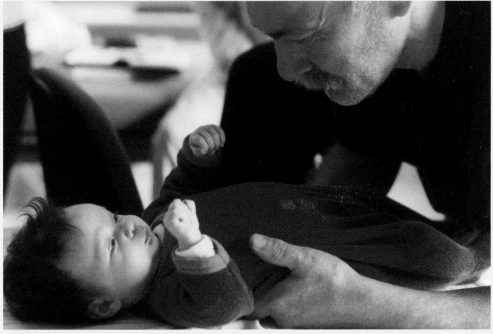

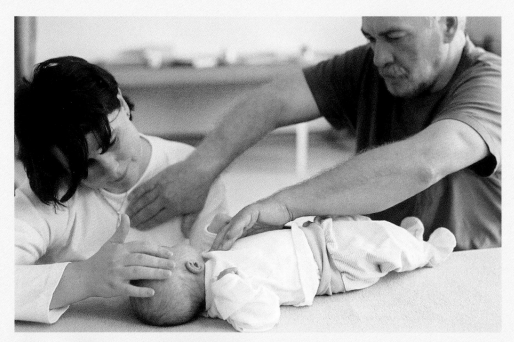

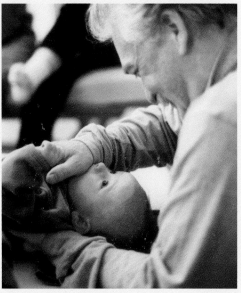

forget that I am connected with the baby and start asking questions to the mother, this almost always brings an immediate protest from the baby.

If contact is not possible because the baby absolutely wants to be with the mother, that is fine with me. After some questions about her experience of the birth process, I give the mother the opportunity to go on the table for a treatment. The connection between them is so deep, and safety for the baby is so important, that I get more by letting the baby feel that what I do is pleasant and good for the mother. Slowly the baby can get used to what I do. Sometimes during the treatment of the mother I will touch the baby, directly or from a distance. This way the little child can slowly get used to my touch.

**CHAPTER 1**

# What Is CS Therapy?

Our body is a perfect self-regulating system. It wakes up and finds its way in the outer world; it lives. At night it sleeps, but what we don't see is the enormous activity in the inside world. Sleep is the time for regeneration, because life wears the cells out. So, in the morning we are fresh and ready to go for another day ... or not. Every form of stress can give us a delay in this repair work, and the body will start functioning a little less perfectly. In our CS treatments we touch the body to feel where the energy is blocked. Those are the places that have been influenced by stress. Compare it with traffic: we look for the traffic jams, make sure that they are cleared ... the therapist is ready!

How does that work? For this you need to know a little about how a body grows. After conception, the egg will clone itself many times until it forms a cluster of exact copies of the original cell. While some of these cells will form the placenta, the rest spread out and form three flat layers, like three pancakes on top of each other. One layer will become the inside, one layer the outside, and one layer the connection between these two. Together these three layers will form our whole body. But near the beginning we are a "short stack" of pancakes consisting of three layers on top of each other.

These pancakes will fold together and form a tube, our primal spinal column. After this, the cells start to migrate to those spots where they will build their own specialized organ and everything else that is inside the body.

To make sure that all works well and that we create a straight house, the first thing that appears in these pancakes is a straight line, the notochord, like a builder's plumb line. This line is like an anchor for every cell and determines and initiates the place and task of every cell. Suddenly all cells know which life task they are going to perform and also where exactly in the body they are going to do that. When they know which organ or brain cell or bone they are going to become, then they start to move and develop in that direction. Once the magic appearance of the notochord delivers its intention, it disappears, but the midline created by the notochord stays always as the dominant direction in our body. Every cell remembers for the rest of its life that original signal which created clarity, which pointed out the right road!

This is one of the basic systems on which our therapy rests: to give back to every cell the trust that comes when you know your life task and the spot on which you can build your own home. We let the person feel, physically, this midline; we place the person precisely in his or her notochord. The natural control mechanism of our body is like a boss giving orders. It makes sure that we eat when it is necessary, that we breathe, digest and do thousands of other things. What we consider to be natural is being done minutely for us by our body. Everybody knows that if you work for a boss and the boss is upset—he/she is full of anxiety or forgot to order something—eventually the whole factory will start feeling the impact of that. Our boss, the brain with its connections, is hidden deep within our body and is being fed and cared for by our CS system. After conception this system grows first and orchestrates the growth of the whole body around itself.

And here we come to the great secret of our therapy. We have learned to feel our boss who is hidden deep within our inside world. We learn to know the nervous system in all its moods. By this feeling we know where problems are and how to solve them. We learn to feel where energy is blocked, release it, and the nervous system can again send its orders without hindrance.

> *When Fidel came for a visit he was five months old. He was shining like the Caribbean sun, so happy, but his breathing was rasping like an old sailor. His mother told me that he had been given asthma medication since he was three months old. After I had him in my arms, I soon felt that in between his shoulder blades, the vertebrae were really pushed on top of each other, which is logical after a heavy birth. Twenty minutes later you could barely hear his breathing. I convinced the mother to use the asthma inhaler only if it was really necessary.*
>
> *Four sessions later Fidel was a healthy baby, his vertebrae were in their natural place, and the nerves that come from the brain and pass in between the vertebrae to give their signals to*

*the lungs were no longer compressed, but free. In short, if the boss has the space to do his work, the body will work just fine.*

Our body, the body that has the wisdom to replace all its worn-out blood cells after a week and to replace itself fully every seven years, without any help, deserves our full respect. Even more remarkable, it is so intelligent that it will tell where it has a problem and also how to solve the problem—at least if you have learned to listen to it.

## CHAPTER 2

# Why Do Babies Need CS Therapy?

To be born we need to re-do the complete evolution. After conception, we are one cell, the impregnated egg. Then, we repeat all the stages from fish to reptile to mammal until we become a human. But it is very difficult to build a house without a proper foundation, so we need to complete every step and if something doesn't fully grow or find its place, we will complete the building of our body on an imperfect base.

After we float like a fish in the amniotic fluid for nine months, the space becomes cramped and we have to get out on dry land. There just isn't enough space inside to grow any further. Coming out is heavy physical labor for mother and child. The soul gets pressed literally into the little body; and in an ideal setting this is done with a natural respect for the timing of the bodies of both mother and child.

The little body is extremely flexible, and the different bones of the skull are like little islands that can move easily. In short, we are like a bag filled with water and a few bones here and there.

The natural quest for life after the baby comes out of the birth canal will unfold the lungs and initiate breathing. The pressure that the lungs put on the spinal column will in turn start the craniosacral (CS) rhythm. This CS rhythm is a strong pumping system for cerebrospinal fluid (CS fluid) within the brain and spinal cord that guarantees the rhythmic opening of the skull and the whole body. The enormous pressure of the occasion of birth, fear of the unknown, and the well-intentioned but sometimes "baby-unfriendly" methods used by the people helping at the delivery can counter the proper unfolding of the little body. Inside the skull there is a certain maximum space available. The more space that is available, the more life energy can fill up this space. But above all, the closer you come to this birth potential, the more space the brain has to grow and do its job.

Our task as CS therapists is to give back all the space that is possible.

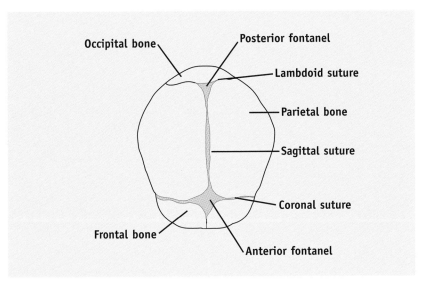

Skull with fontanels.

The top of the head must be used as a battering ram to go through the birth canal, passing the pelvic bones. The bones of the head each have two or more moving parts with sutures and fontanels to accommodate these narrow passageways and be able to go with the flow.

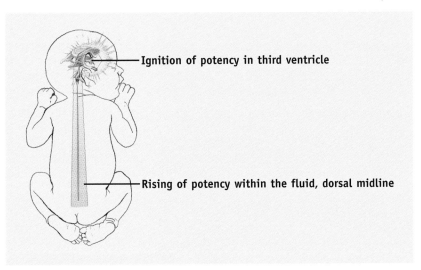

"Ignition."

"Ignition" is Franklyn Sills' expression for the life force that awakens in the baby. That is how our lives begin ... if we get a chance.

## Where to Expect Problems?

The physical problems arise when the unfolding of the little body cannot be completed. The strong compression and de-compression forces will move the little bones over each other during birth, and if they get stuck, nerves or blood vessels can become blocked.

The most vulnerable spot is of course the skull (and neck) because of its use as a battering ram to force its way out, or its use as a lever to be pulled out of the birth canal. Furthermore, the spinal column can become compressed and twisted.

Problems that arise, and about which the baby will voice its displeasure strongly, have to do with systems or organs that do not get enough space to do their job because of all this pressure.

Usually the baby will solve most of these pressure problems itself. Via breastfeeding it will develop so much sucking power that parts of the "snout" and the skull will break loose from each other and find their own natural spot. If this self-help program isn't enough, we can mostly dispatch these compressions in a few sessions.

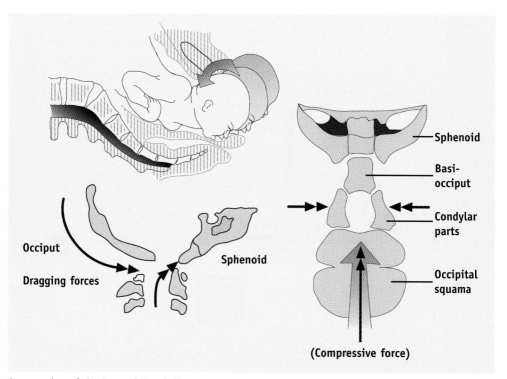

Compression of the base of the skull.

### Cranial Bones Can Slide Over Each Other During Birth

You can compare the little head with a bag filled with water. The very flexible and moveable bones of the skull are solidifications of that bag and are not yet fully grown. That's the reason why very big spaces (fontanels) separate those bones. Slight bending of these bones and sliding over each other are normal and necessary to come through the birth canal.

Only when some of these bones stay stuck on top of each other will it prevent the growth of the brain and so impede, sometimes dramatically, the workings of the body. Of course as CS therapists we will do our best to make sure that these overlaps are corrected.

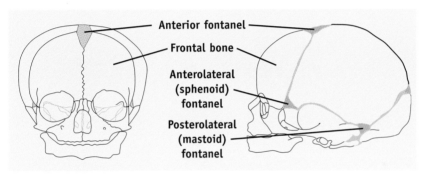

The little bones can slide over each other when necessary.

The **frontal bone** consists of two parts.
The **sphenoid** consists of three parts.
The **temporal bone** consists of three parts.
The **occiput** consists of four parts.
The **ethmoid** consists of three parts.
The **maxilla** (upper jaw) consists of two parts.
The **mandible** (lower jaw) consists of two parts.
The **atlas** consists of three parts.
The **sacrum** consists of five parts.

The most vulnerable spot is the base of the skull. Here, nerves and blood vessels go in and out of the skull, and in the middle is that very thick bunch of nerves that we call the spinal column. A very well-known nerve that can become easily irritated there is the vagus nerve. It regulates the function of almost all organs as well as the breathing and digestion and the relaxation of the heart. Furthermore, there is a nerve at the base of the skull that relaxes or tenses the muscles of the neck, and this becomes an extra difficulty if this nerve is compressed.

Most of these nerves have strong connections with each other, and compressions give rise to cumulative problems.

Of course our body will adapt and learn to live with dysfunctions but it isn't the most happy start possible, as every parent of a crybaby will tell you. All these little problems can (amongst others) lead to hyperactive behavior, which can be a hell on earth, and the child doesn't even know the source of the discomfort and can't communicate about it.

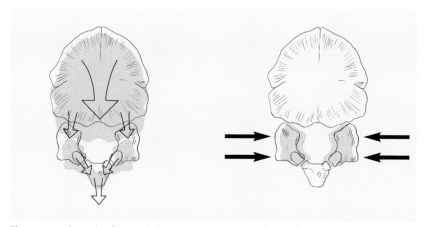

The arrows show the forces that can compress the spinal column.
Without corrections this will lead to hyperactive behavior.

## CHAPTER 3

# Our Survival Strategies Concerning Birth and Their Influence on Our Life

Let me make one thing clear: almost all problems that arise during birth can be resolved through love. However heavy and threatening birth can be, the bonding process with the mother will make up for most of these problems. If more is needed, a few CS treatments can solve almost all problems. Untreated, our first experiences will determine or at least influence our behavior for the rest of our lives. Being born is how we promote the survival of our species; and in our bodies, defense mechanisms are present that will start working shortly after conception to maintain this survival. At birth they take their place and are fully active.

A newly-born is totally unable to look after itself, and the development of different, higher brain functions will take years to complete. So for survival, the help of the mother needs to be guaranteed, and for this, the little body has a choice of three different scenarios.* Let's look at it from the outside in, from the most developed to the most primitive.

1. The most developed part of our brain that is available after birth is the **mammalian brain**, but mother and child need to have an opportunity to activate it. The hormonal bonding that gets activated will guarantee a safe and satisfied feeling for the mother and her baby. This way, survival of the species and the individual is guaranteed.

    If you look at a mother and her baby during breastfeeding you can literally see the cocoon around them during these most intimate times. Touch and soft sounds and smells that accompany this interaction reveal love right in front of your eyes. It is of course evident that the breasts of the mother sit exactly on top of her heart, so the baby enjoys liquid love as food!

---

* Paul MacLean was the first to describe the "triune brain model" about the threefold compilation of the brain. (Paul D. MacLean, *The Triune Brain in Evolution.* NY: Plenum Press, 1990.) As I describe this compilation, the terminology is a little more simple.

This intimacy is necessary to activate the hormonal bonding system, and the most decisive factor required to turn on this hormonal switch is breastfeeding. If for any reason the baby is taken away for all kinds of tests or the mother needs to be treated, then the baby will be forced to use older evolutionary defense mechanisms.

2. The **reptilian brain** (the sympathetic nervous system) lies literally under the mammalian brain.

   Activation of the reptilian brain, because the higher mammalian brain wasn't switched on, will produce stress hormones in mother and child. For an adult this brain activates a fight/flight mechanism, but for a baby, screaming is the only way to express itself and ensure that it will get the full attention from its surroundings. This way the mother's fight/flight mechanism becomes active. Screaming out of frustration, disappointment or pain will make sure that the mother reacts via the production of her own stress hormones. The sound of such a baby will almost always get the same reaction in everybody in the neighborhood, and that is the purpose of this brain in the baby.

3. In extreme circumstances, if the first and second layers don't function, the still older **worm-like brain** (the parasympathetic nervous system) will become active and the baby will become completely passive.

The differentiation of the brain in layers that are stacked on top of one another is the result of the way in which we had to deal with new circumstances and challenges of the evolving world around us—the only way to survive was to evolve ourselves. Every new layer of our brain developed some more possibilities to exceed that of the brain as it was before. New strategies needed new and more complicated wiring in their guidance systems.

It is these three systems stacked on top of each other that will guarantee our survival. If one of these systems hasn't been activated there is always an older, underlying but consequently more primitive system to fall back on. Just like that time when you needed to go to work but your car didn't want to start. Your bicycle had a flat tire, so you decided to go on foot . . . or did you call in sick? Some of us even keep on doing this chronically.

The difficulties that can arise in those survival strategies will often determine our lifetime patterns. Feeling safe and secure will be guaranteed if the mammalian brain is activated; if not, then there is always a subconscious fear about our survival. Life becomes almost impossible if you end up in the lethargic world under that, a world without emotions, because you were unable to activate any of your higher possibilities. We all remember images of those Romanian orphanages with those empty-eyed babies and small children.

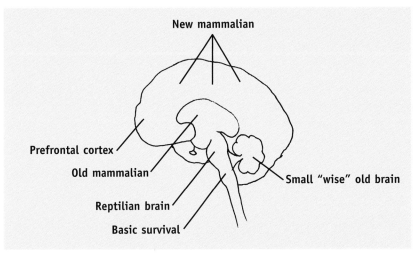

Every new development gives us a few more possibilities to function at a higher level.

All these basic systems will start developing during conception or sometime during pregnancy and will consider their first stress level as their neutral position. Those with too-highly stressed starting points can experience enormous behavioral disturbances that are positioned just under conscious awareness ... like a layer cake. In other words, one often doesn't know where some fear or discomfort or dreams come from, because they have always been there.

If the emotional bonding (mammalian brain) doesn't happen, it remains a hiatus in your development. You will always search for this bonding but at the same time you won't know how to make the connection. This is, for example, the case with the man (or woman) who looks for his mother in every female.

Try to put a roof on top of walls that are crooked because the foundation is missing something. In our practice we often see that it is impossible for some clients to find balance in their lives because one of their basic needs hasn't been met. If you look at this step-by-step progression in human behavior, the impossibility for peace in some parts of the world becomes understandable. Imagine that you are growing in a womb and you can hear and feel bombs falling and exploding, and the stress hormones that go with that become your day-to-day reality!

In our therapy with grown-ups we see innumerable behavioral disturbances arising from the womb, and luckily it is still possible to correct most of them.

### Our Newest Achievement and Hope for the Future

On top of the three aforementioned brains, with the worm-like brain as the oldest, sits a filter. This filter, the thalamus, decides for itself what is allowed to penetrate into our consciousness, including physical impulses as well as psychological issues. It will not allow problems into your consciousness which it knows you are not ready to deal with.

The prefrontal cortex (just above the sphenoid) is the place where we become conscious of our selves. It is our last development. It creates scenarios for future use and is our window into the future—how we can influence the future. This place uses the bulk of our energy because we can never stop devising plans.

Joseph Chilton Pearce* connects another brain to this, the transforming brain, the heart (as a brain). Sixty percent of our heart tissue is made of neurons, which are connected with the brain, especially the prefrontal cortex. That's why the heart has a very big influence on the working of our brain and thus on brain energy. What does a heart do with all that energy? Transforms it. Because of this we have the capacity to connect with the outside world in a totally new way, with a compassionate mind.

The stacking of our different brains with the heart as the transforming factor fits in perfectly with the Chinese concept of the "triple-heater," which also describes our energy's topography. The first level of the triple-heater is a spot just under the navel, the *hara*, that

---

* Joseph Chilton Pearce, *The Biology of Transcendence: A Blueprint of the Human Spirit* (Rochester, VT: Park Street Press, 2002).

contains the energy with which we are born. This energy keeps our soul connected to this body and gives rise to its form.

The second spot sits just under our pelvic diaphragm; here all the organs that digest food and provide our daily doses of energy are situated. It makes sure that we stay alive and maintain our form.

The third part of the triple-heater is the heart. The heart transforms all this energy in such a way that it can be understood and used by the body, and so communication with the outside world can happen. It gives us the possibility to connect again to the whole.

For both energies, physical and mental, the heart is the connecting factor. This is remarkable and shows us clearly our life path. Our heart is the physical connecting factor and the only power on Earth strong enough to calm down the tyranny of the mind. Communication via the heart gives the mind time to rest, so that it can become fresh with new ideas and can become active with new possibilities when that is necessary.

## SERIES 2 - Little Man

This session is shown as it is done. There is no protocol. I just follow what the body asks me to do.

These two places are asking for contact.

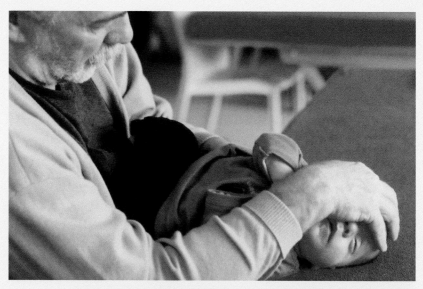

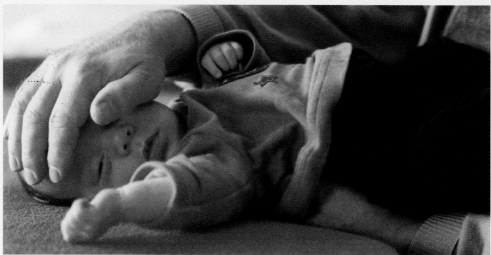

The little body shows me clearly that the head at the front is stuck. And at the back, exactly where my hand is, I can feel the vertebrae are stuck on top of one another.

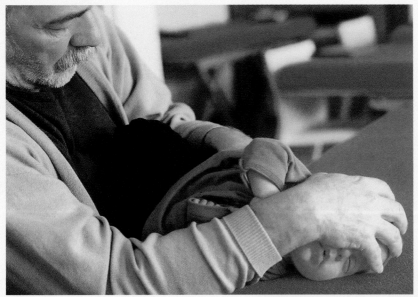

The cell memories are getting stronger
and are asking gravity for help.

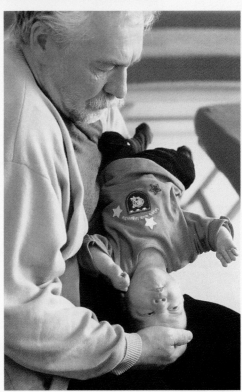

Off the table, body to body, the feeling of
the birth canal is very close by.

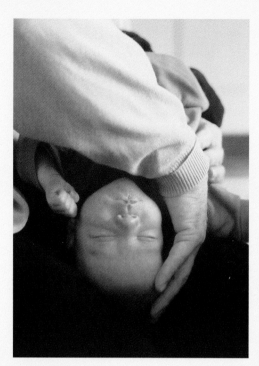

This is a good moment to have a little rest.

Here we go again. Softly the head glides off my hand as if it is passing the pubic bone.

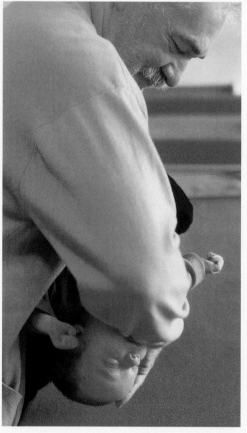

The head that is touching my hand becomes lighter and the flow towards the navel opens up.

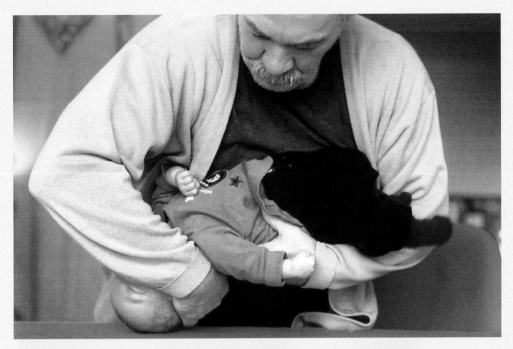

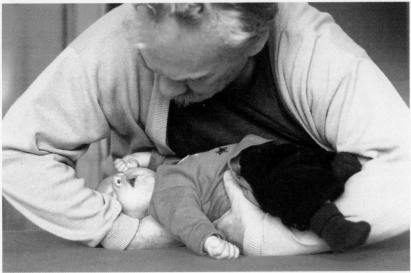

I am monitoring the flow of the fluid that is pushing the atlas and occiput apart, and I am acknowledging its movement towards the sacrum; it is a flow that brings quietness and clarity.

The solution: space ... the head lightens up.

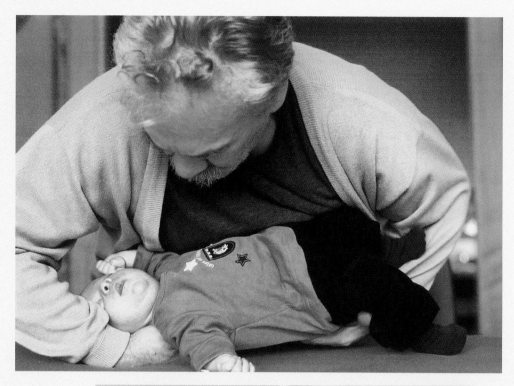

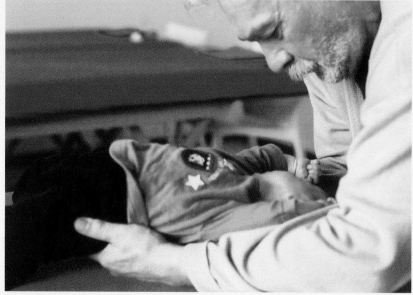

The result: total surrender in a vibrating still-point.

Unwinding of parts of the occiput, we are still in a quiet spot and EV4 is announcing itself.

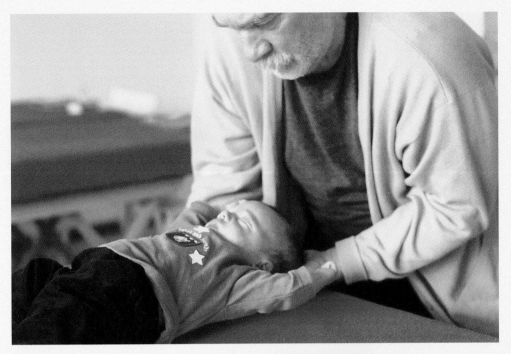

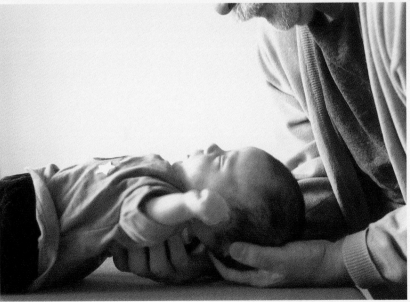

Re-alignment is happening with a little help from my fingers.

Spreading of the condyles while I release the fascia of the trapezius.

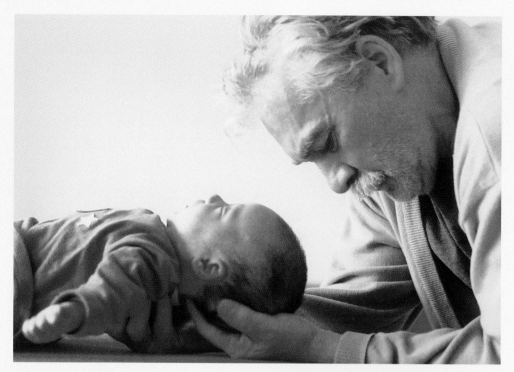

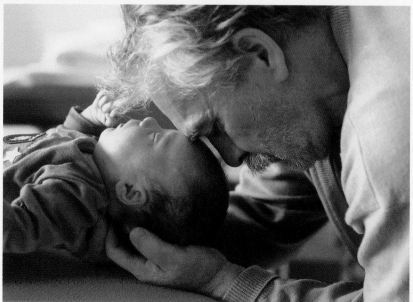

Unity.

The head turns a little to show me a compression around the bottom of the temporal bone connected with C2 and C3.

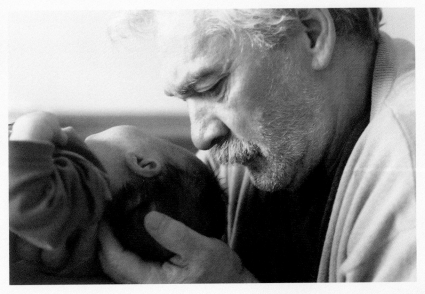

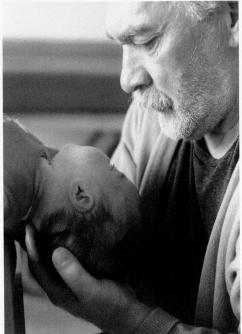

The occiput elongates and the turbine in the third ventricle lightens up.

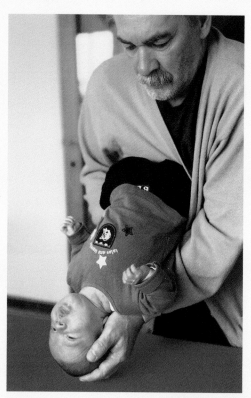

All babies are from the very beginning Buddhas. A unique being emerges.

Just another stretch.

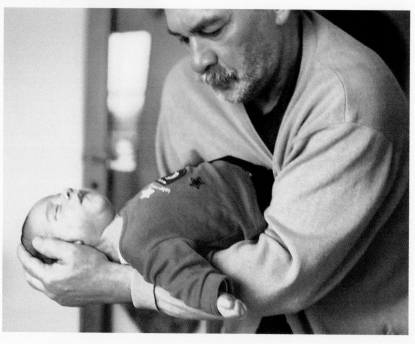

**Craniosacral Therapy for Babies and Small Children**

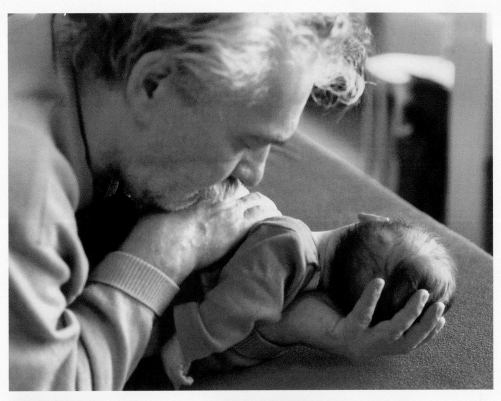

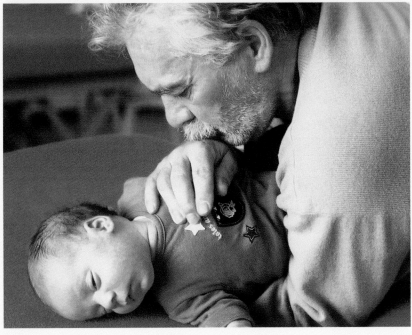

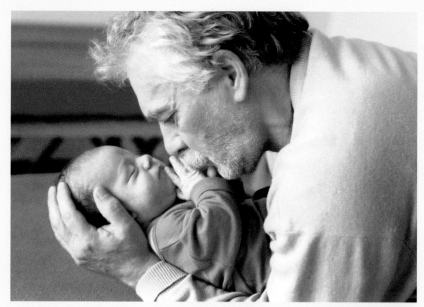

Love heals.

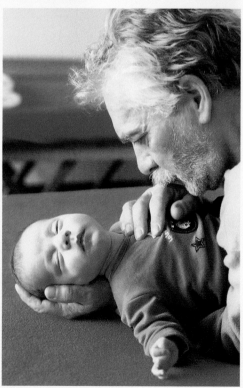

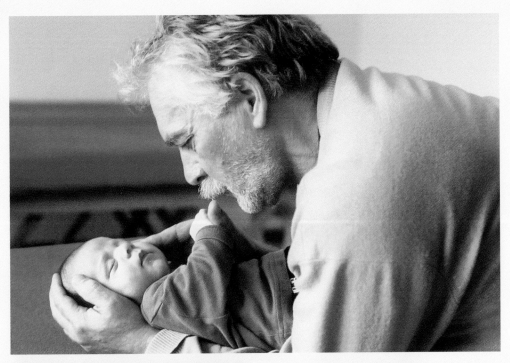

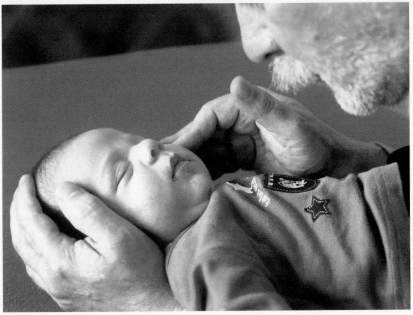

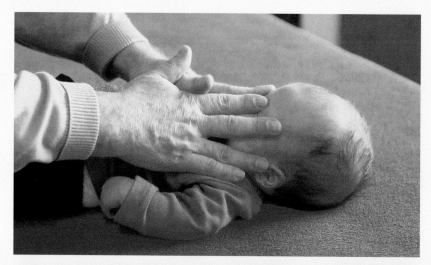

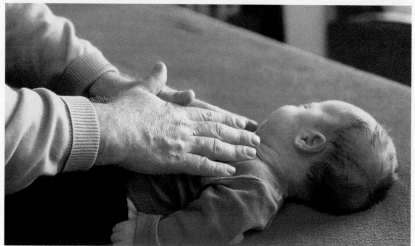

"Listen, little man, let me show you how gravity works."

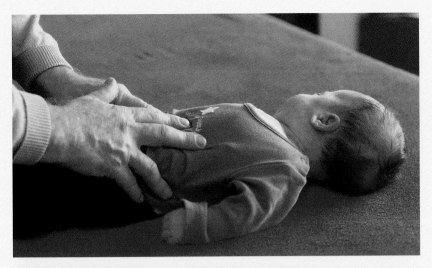

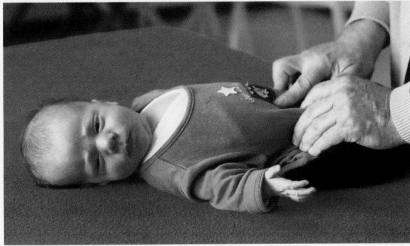

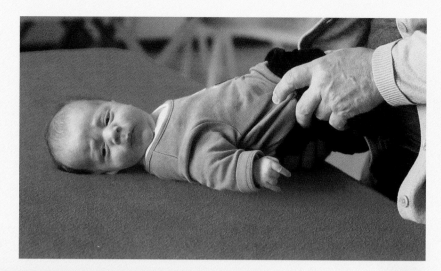

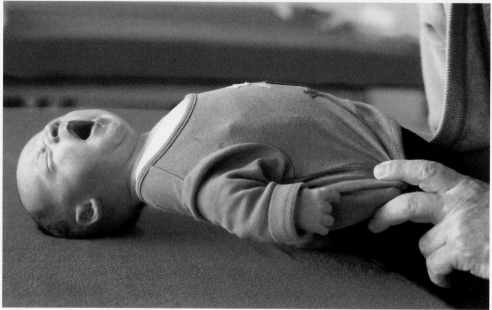

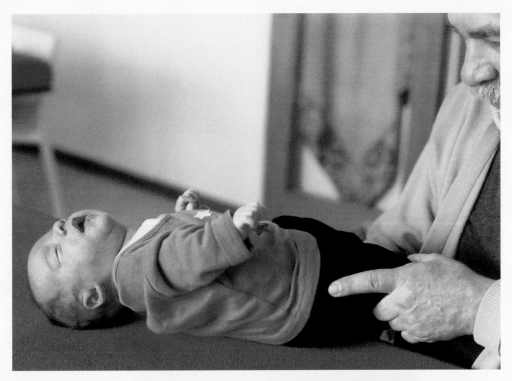

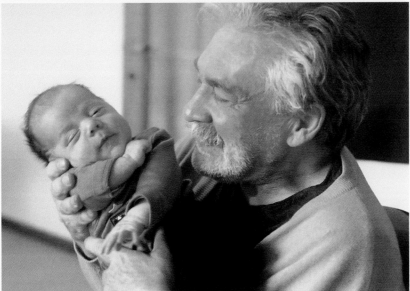

We thank each other.

## CHAPTER 4

# About a Love Cocktail and the Creation of a Hormonal Womb

At birth everything is present, but few things in the body can be used because only the simplest mechanisms are working.

We've had millions of years to perfect the scenario that will connect mother and baby to each other, and the production of the love hormones such as oxytocin will play a major role. During labor, the mother's body also produces an enormous amount of endorphins to relieve most of the pain, and these endorphins will circulate within the body for a while as well. The combination of both hormones creates a potent love cocktail, and some women cannot get enough of this. This chemical bond between mother and child will satisfy our primal wish for survival. It guarantees the baby that the mother cannot do anything else but feel love for it; and the woman, whether she wishes it or not, will change into a mother!

Nevertheless we, in our "supreme wisdom," will do everything in our power to make this primal bond as difficult as possible . . . indeed, there is nothing easier than to take the child away just after birth for a whole bunch of tests, eye drops, weighing, etc. (that cannot be done later?), and so those very important hormones cannot manifest properly and do their job fully and naturally.

It is in this phase, when mother and child need to create a "hormonal womb," that every interference by technical specialists can cause disruptions and interferences with the natural process. And it is even possible that the woman doesn't get a chance to transform into a mother. This can be a contributing cause of postnatal depression. The birth protocol created by the hospital does not take this necessary bond into sufficient account, and it is here that evolution can lose its grounding.

For all clarity: this hormonal womb is the bond that will bind mother and child externally. This "honeymoon," this bonding process between mother and child, will last from twelve to sixteen months.

## Getting Born You Never Do Alone!

The emotional bond between mother and child can only be complete if both get a chance to produce the appropriate hormones. Only then can one say that not only a child but also a mother was born.

Problems that can arise for the baby are connected with the very heavy birth process where we are literally pressed into our body. When we come out of our mother's belly after a very exhausting time, our new body has to find the strength to unfold completely and, by doing so, create the necessary space to make itself function maximally. This complete compression of the skull is of course a little frightening, but don't forget, that's the way it is supposed to be; and that's the way mammals have been arriving for millions of years. It is not always a blessing that we as humans are the most advanced species. Especially in the last century we have been leading sedentary lives, and as a result, our bodies have lost their natural flexibility and strength. This advanced way of life ensures that we humans are the only species on Earth that needs assistance in the birth process. But don't worry, as an intelligent species we have learned to cope with this, and it gives us CS therapists a fine opportunity to help with something enormously space-giving. Believe me, there is nothing more satisfying than to look a new soul in the eyes and to free up its physical blocks and give it the space that it needs.

The theft of the birth ritual by the obstetrical caste and the many "Dr. Spocks," with their birth and education schemes and baby formulae instead of mother's milk, have pushed the whole country (USA and many others) into the sympathetic defense mechanism. According to Joseph Chilton Pearce, in the USA at one time 97% of babies were raised with bottle-feeding—in other words, everybody. And breastfeeding is key to activating the mammalian brain!

An activated mammalian brain makes it possible for our prefrontal cortex (the human brain) to develop on a firm emotional base. This instrument of natural creativity can investigate the world in a free and open manner. If you put your own ideas of how the world is into the new mind of the baby early enough, it will lose its freedom to investigate in an unhindered way, and creativity and the ability for self-reflection disappear. Religious education does exactly that. It puts somebody else's car in your garage, and if you hear often enough that it is your car, you believe it. If you do these things on top of a not fully activated mammalian brain, then you create the problems that the world knows today: crusading for democracy, jihad, and in the face of HIV/AIDS, "a condom is not God's will." It becomes unlikely that a person will be able to decipher the difference between what is true and what is propaganda. It also is easy to see how warlike responses to a national trauma may look like the only path of choice.

## Treatment

The principle of treatment for a not-fully-activated mammalian brain and thus a fully activated autonomic system (both the reptilian and worm-like brain) is quite simple to explain. The energy (the soul) that incarnates and will express itself in a human form will do so from the center of the body outwards. This center, completely in the middle of the body, is the place where the CS fluid circulates (also called the cerebrospinal fluid). The CS fluid is the primary recipient of this energy, which is pure, and in essence, "unity." And therefore it will always carry in itself the memory of unity. When this energy starts expressing itself in a form, in matter (by the constraints of space) it will start to shine outwards in order to reach its maximum potential.

With a natural birth, when the original energy is able to express itself to the max, it will activate one by one every system until finally the mammalian brain, with its hormonal workings (and thus the formation of the hormonal womb) will be the natural result.

If the system isn't fully activated, the body will have to be content with the underlying sympathetic or the even lower parasympathetic system. Therefore if one of those systems is stuck, change can only come from the inside, from the center. Recognizing and "potentializing" that basic energy will push away all surrounding obstacles. By reinforcing it with "intent," the memory of the fluid with its own power will become stronger. The slowest CS rhythm is the place where we can connect to this power most deeply and let it flow outwards.

All obstacles will be pushed outwards through this power, and frustrations, fear, anger and all primal emotions will need to be expressed. Only then can the baby allow again the refinement of its basic energy and claim its birthright. The different brains can then become activated.

**Only then can love be experienced and named.**

## CHAPTER 5

# Guideline for the Treatment of Mother and Child after Birth

- When a baby is brought to me, I start the treatment as soon as the baby feels safe with me, sometimes in the hands of its mother or safe in its maxicozy. Once the session starts I maintain eye contact with this new life. This is a most important thing; the energy that is transmitted through the eyes will replace the old contact, the umbilical cord.

- Asking permission is not always necessary, especially not aloud; eye contact, very slow movements and sounds will make that permission automatic.

- If you need to talk, then do it slowly and softly. If you need to ask a question, then do this slowly and wait for the answer—it will come one way or another. Remember this little body is so new that it will have to create new neurons in order to give you an answer.

- How would you feel if people talked about you in your own presence as though you were not there? So never talk to somebody else when you are working with a baby. Your touch and attention need to be total.

- There is nothing that you have to do; the body of the baby will tell you what can happen and has to happen. Every baby is a Zen master, so enjoy its presence.

- If one of the defense mechanisms is not in its neutral position, then this needs to be restored. It will often be accompanied with a letting go of frustrations. Love (=unity=bonding) will dissolve almost all sympathetic and parasympathetic problems.

- If during the treatment an insecure situation arises for the baby, the mother needs to be involved before you can go on; what is empty or threatened needs to be filled with love (=security).

- If the baby doesn't want what is happening or if there is some doubt, ask the mother to go on the table and treat her, sometimes with the baby on her belly and its head on her heart. Mother is so under the influence of "caring-for" hormones that she might forget to look after herself. With the baby on top of her, she will usually full-heartedly agree to be treated. When she starts to relax under your hands, you can also start touching the baby, if need be from a distance.

- Mothers who get enough nurturing and attention from their partners will be able to devote themselves fully to their changed designation; on top of that, breastfeeding will regulate their own hormonal workings.

- Pelvic instability can arise and can be treated by the known CS pelvic techniques. When it happens before labor, there is often an emotional component that needs to be investigated.

- I advise new mothers to be treated once a month, according to their circumstances.

> *I will never forget baby Anton. He was two weeks old. While I was touching him and asking questions to the mother about the labor, I got quite a shock when I looked into his eyes. Then the world, my world, stood still. His world was slow and quiet and there was absolutely no mind present. There was only openness and silent innocence. Since then, if I don't forget, I always start with looking into the baby's eyes and letting him/her look back into mine, absorbing its smell and only then touching its body. I will talk very slowly and very quietly, just a whisper in its ear. If you have been received then you will see the baby's whole body relax. The hands will open and the arms will stop all movement. And, perhaps even more importantly, you will receive that gentle energy back from the baby and the dimension from which it has come. It came as a revelation to me that babies also want and need to give love back. I was able to receive it with so much gratitude.*

## CHAPTER 6

# The Different Techniques

### Touching the Sacrum

The sacrum is a good place to start. The ascending energy out of my hand is, to the body, comparable to the energy which was moving upwards via the umbilical cord. The sacrum is a safe place for the baby and a good place for us to listen to the body. It is the base on which the rest of the body can rest.

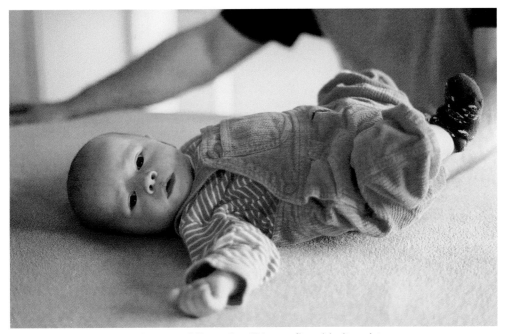

By carrying the baby in a "haptonomic" way, it will be confirmed in its existence. It happens when you put a hand under the sacrum to carry, touch or lift a baby.

### Freeing Up the Spine

While the baby is coming out, compression forces can push the vertebrae on top of one another. The nerves that come out from between the vertebrae will be compressed, which will result in diminished function of the related organs. A lot of breathing problems will be relieved by decompressing these vertebrae. The corkscrew motion that the baby's body needs to make to come out of the body of the mother can cause twists in the spinal and brain meninges, and also in the bones of the spine, the pelvis or head. When you create a driveway to get into your garage, you want to make sure this route is as straight as it can be so you can get into and out of your garage as easily as possible. Luckily after all the violence of the birth process, there is a chance to straighten out the road between body and brain so that traffic jams can be avoided in the future.

### Treatment

Let your hands hold both ends of the dura mater (the occiput and the sacrum). Then wait until you both become silent. The rotation patterns will show themselves, and there is nothing else to do but follow these. Out of this technique comes the invitation to go into "no-time." This is the sphere from which the baby has come, the sphere in which the baby created its own body. With the enormous slowness that is necessary, we wait now in order to allow the rotations to lift themselves. The intention towards the sacrum together with the CS fluid directed towards the head can be reinforced by gravity.

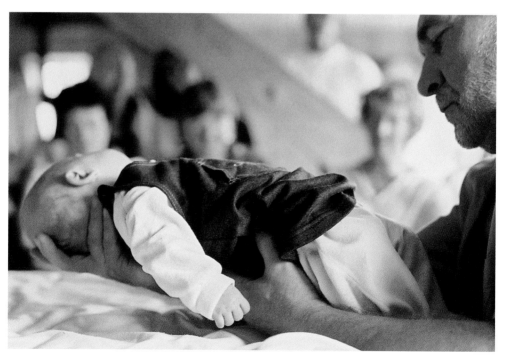

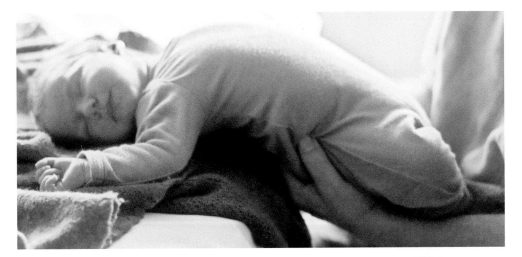

The intention of gravity is the force that helps create our body. It is this force that will trap cosmic energy here on Earth and force it to express itself in a physical form. By the grace of gravity we can be born. Gravity is also an essential factor in the way the soul enters into matter.

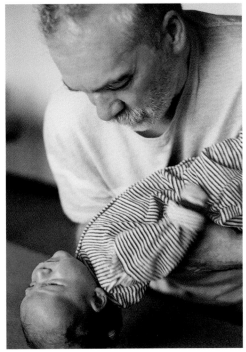

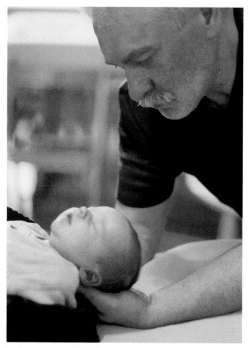

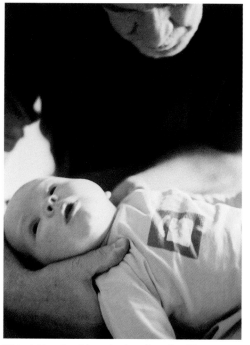

Releasing CV4 by slight pressure, obstacles will be pushed away.

EV4 at the shoulders: by keeping the CS system open, you invite potency into the CS fluid.

## Compression and Expansion Techniques: CV4 and EV4

CV4 can be used when the base of the skull, the occiput, has been compressed too much. The CV4 technique is done by compressing the fourth ventricle. Let the occiput rest on the pads of your thumbs while your hands are cradled. Once your hands relax, you can feel the CS rhythm; follow this rhythm when it moves to the midpoint and on its deepest point you almost equal the pressure. This way you get a higher pressure within the CS fluid, which will have a correcting and cleansing effect inside the total dura mater.

The technique I describe is how it should be done in adults; with babies I sometimes use two fingers of one hand, sometimes two hands, but to do this on a baby, one needs special sensitivity and a lot of practice on adults. **In order to avoid damage, let me repeat, this technique should be used only after years of practice.**

Compression techniques at the shoulders or the pelvis have to do with the specific way that the baby came through the birth canal. They are "follow" techniques, where the compression that you feel is confirmed and encouraged. You just wait for the reverse motion; you wait until the body tells you that there is enough power in the system for the compression to be pushed out. This technique is usually followed by the EV4 technique.

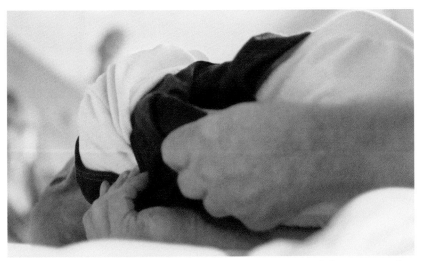

Compressing and holding the vertebrae forces a correction around the sacrum and hip joint.

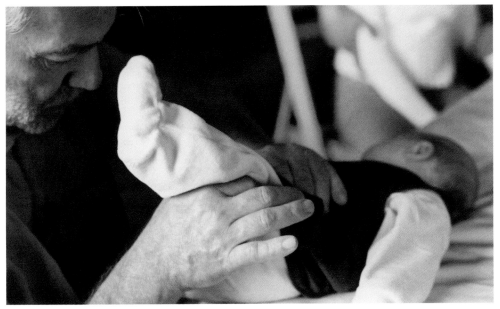

The leg slowly places itself in the hip joint.

EV4 is a technique by which the CS system can be held open fully. It is an invitation for the cosmic life-force to enter into the CS fluid and activate it maximally. When you follow the CS rhythm and the shoulders are in their almost maximum expansion mode, you keep them there. You notice that your arms follow an opening direction; you clearly are inviting something into the CS fluid of your client. If you don't hold this expansion too tight, but allow a little movement in this extreme position, you will feel that the fluid gets an "enlightened" quality.

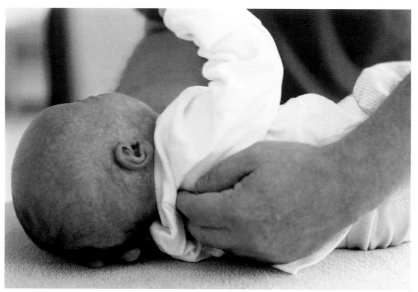

I am compressing the shoulders to release fascia and the bones involved to elongate the spine.

### Creating Space When Bones of the Skull are Overlapping

The bones of a baby's head are not fully formed and they are like little islands growing towards each other. Between the bones exist big fontanels. This allows a lot of movement and even the possibility of overrides, making our journey through the birth canal easier. After birth, the power inside the CS system will make sure that the overriding bones get back to their most ideal place. Sometimes though, they stay stuck on top of each other and this limits growing space for the brain. The sutures in the middle, from front to back and from ear to ear, may ride over each other. The part of the brain that sits there is responsible for a lot of our motion, and lack of space can cause spasticity.

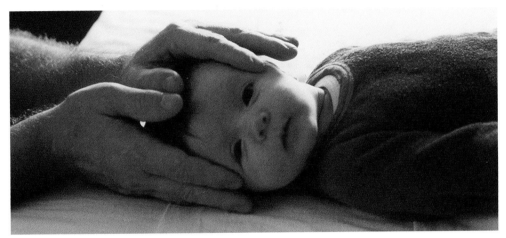

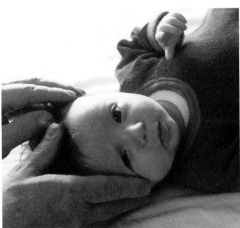

The hands are next to each other on the bones that have an override.

---

### Treatment

With **intention**\* you move the bones apart by holding each bone with one or two fingers while you send energy to that spot from the opposite side of the head and/or occiput.

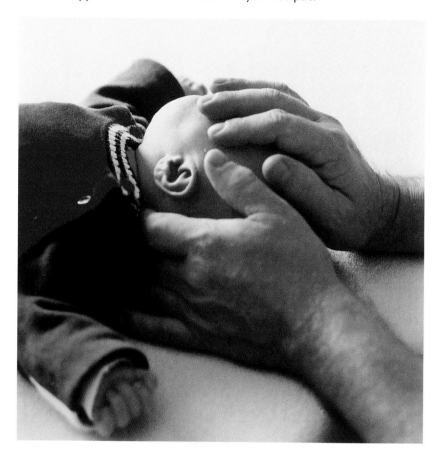

---

\* Intention connects your own energy and power with cosmic influences. The more cosmic energy that you can allow, the finer, more direct and clearer your own energy and intention get.

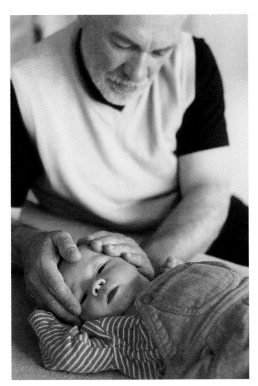 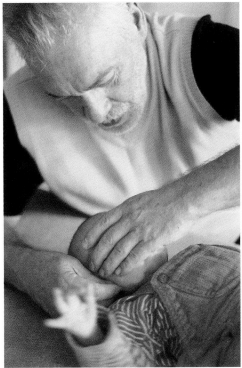

The same compression forces that push bones on top of each other you often feel in one bone, because it feels thicker and compressed. To release this tension you work in the same way. Place your fingers around this spot and give the bones the feeling that expansion is possible. If you can, send energy and the idea of space to that spot from the opposite side of the head. Time, silence, and intention will always create space.

## Ear Techniques

The temporal bones are in three parts during birth, and the opening between temporal bone and occiput will always have to deal with compression forces and twists. At the base of the skull, cranial nerves that use the opening between occiput and temporal bone to exit the skull (vagus, hypoglossal, glossopharyngeal, spinal accessory) can become severely blocked, as can the blood flow going into and exiting the skull. In babies, problems with digestion (like colic), impairment of the sucking reflex, and breathing problems can arise. In adult life this can lead to migraines, digestive problems, breathing problems, tinnitus, chronic fatigue, low potency, and hearing and learning disabilities.

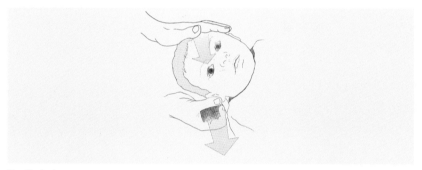

Ear Technique

### Treatment

If sideways expansion of the tentorium* via the two ears is not possible, you take hold of one ear while the other hand rests diagonally above the opposite eye. Direct energy towards and slightly under the ear where your fingertips make contact. Follow the movements and slowly replace them by a movement that gives freedom to the bones. Do this with both ears and take time to balance yourself via the ears of the baby, as if the hand on top holds the string and the ear is the weight of the pendulum, slowly unwinding.

---

\* The tent (tentorium) is the horizontal meninges that divides the inside of the skull into two levels. Under the tent on the lowest level you find the cerebellum, and on the first floor above the tent you find the cerebrum. There is also another meninges, the falx, that divides the inside of the skull into a left and a right space. The combination of all these meninges ensures that the skull is divided into four separate spaces, with an opening for the older brain parts in the middle (medulla, pons, and limbic system, which are other terms for the worm-like, reptilian, and mammalian brain).

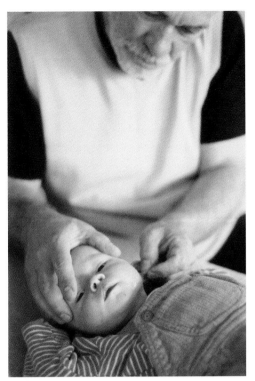

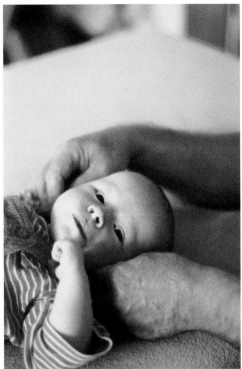

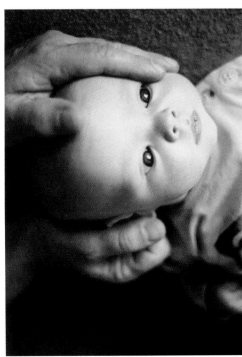

### Finger in the Mouth Technique Using the Sucking Reflex

Sucking is a natural reflex and enables the baby to take food for the first time independently. Not only is food being taken in, but the sucking power will influence the hard palate in such a way that it will optimize the working of the CS system. Breasts grow on top of the heart, and when a baby sucks, he or she receives liquid love from the mother. In the body of the mother, the sucking of the baby will shrink the uterus and bring it back to its ideal size and place. Sucking at the breast tells the organs in the belly of the mother that they have achieved their life task and that they can rest for a while, and it will also act as a natural contraceptive. All these effects of breastfeeding guarantee survival of the baby, maximize the baby's immune system, and realign the reproductive organs of the mother; and in order to accomplish this, nature makes sure that it is an orgasmic experience.

> *In my work I sometimes treat women with breast cancer. It is my feeling that a lot of these cancers arise when the breasts didn't fulfill their life task; it seems the cells just become disgusted or so frustrated that they create a cancer. This is not only my point of view; it is reported to be the case in countless sessions I have had with breast-cancer patients.*

With this technique of the finger in the baby's mouth, we simply bring on the sucking reflex. It gives us a way to maximize the CS rhythm if that is necessary, and it also gives us a good handle to correct bones that are not in their right position.

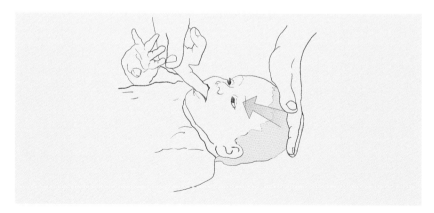

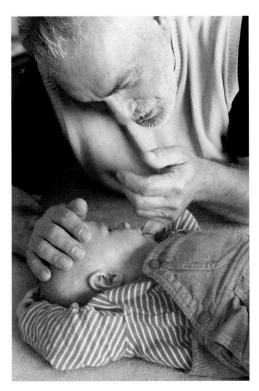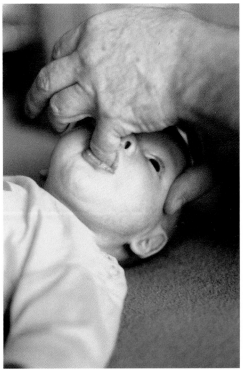

One of my grandchildren was born with a slightly crooked nose, and because of that, one eye was a little higher than the other. As usual, the parents did notice, but went into denial and it was soon blocked out. On top of that, our daughter-in-law was so protective that we were only allowed to touch the baby in their presence. One evening we were allowed to babysit (it took the parents eighteen minutes to come back). Of course I just couldn't resist putting my finger in the baby's mouth so it could suck, while I convinced the bones softly to get back to their optimal spots. When the parents returned, my son asked, "Did you do something?" I said, "Why should I?" No word was said about it, nothing was ever mentioned again, and our grandchild's head is perfect!

**Treatment**

Make sure that your hands are washed and that your nails are clipped. Tickle a little at the side of the mouth until the sucking reflex begins. Put your finger in the mouth and make contact with the hard palate and the vomer. Let your finger move with every movement that happens until you feel some balance. Place the other hand on top of the head or on the sphenoid until you can make a connection between both hands. Your intention will potentialize the vomer, which you follow until the vomer radiates power.

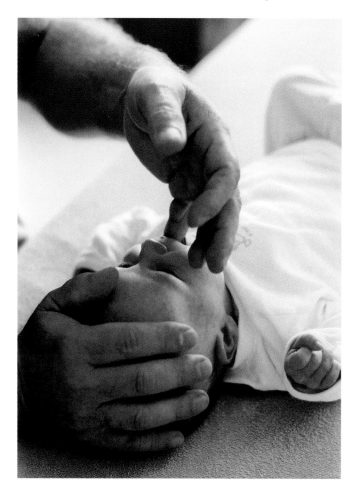

## Atlas/Occiput Technique

By its special structure this place is the most vulnerable and is also responsible for very unpleasant problems, like hyperkinetic (a.k.a. hyperactive) behavior. The occiput at birth is still in four different pieces that encompass the spinal column. Compression forces will always push this region together, and to top it off, this is the spot around which the little head will bend if the head cannot find an easy exit. Every disturbance, even minimal, can disrupt the working of the organs or the signals that need to arrive to the brain. On the bottom of the occiput there are two little knobs that can become stuck on top of the first vertebra, the atlas. The four loose parts of the occiput will start growing together in the first year after birth, and if you don't intervene, this place, due to the compression forces, will be too narrow for all the traffic that needs to come by every moment of the day.

We all know the impossible irritations that can arise at roadblocks, and this is exactly a spot like that, but on the main cross-section of the body. All decisions that are made in the head about the workings of the body, and everything that the body feels and needs to send to the head to make correct decisions, have to pass through this opening. If this spot is too narrow the irritations are there, but this you don't wish on any child. A baby that has to deal with these problems has no other solution than to voice its discomfort and pain, hoping that somebody can do something; their screaming is a deep cry for help! Breathing problems, sucking and feeding problems, colic and diarrhea are all indications that there is not enough space for every nerve to send its signal.

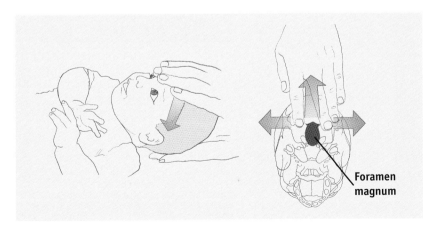

Foramen magnum

**Treatment**

The techniques that we know are very specialized, and if you start treating before the parts are fused together, the result will be easier to reach and more complete.

1. Hold the head at the base and take your time to relax so that you can feel the flow in the head. A soft sideways spreading will arise by itself. Your intention is directed to the spreading out of the center of the occiput.

2. When necessary you can do the spreading out with one hand while the other hand sends energy from the frontal towards your fingertips.

3. Accept and confirm all movements that you feel in the bone, let them come to rest, and initiate a movement that is necessary to bring everything again into the middle; the feeling of space and lightness will arise.

4. The occiput is now ready to move out of its compression towards you.

5. Let your hands maintain the contact until you and the bones and the baby can come to rest in this new freedom.

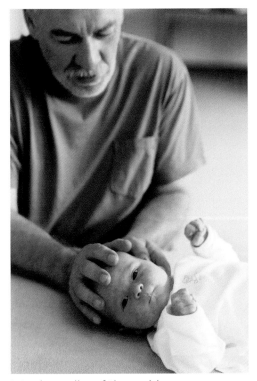
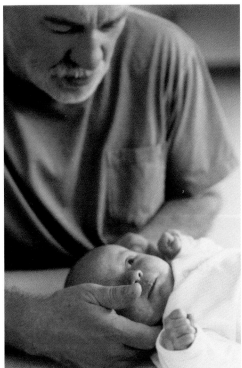

Lateral spreading of the condyles.

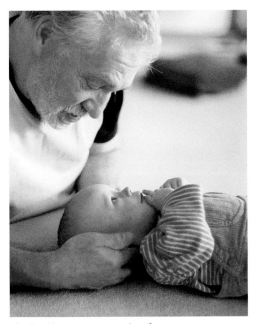

The backbone starts coming free.

## Sphenoid Technique

The sphenoid is placed so centrally in the head that it can be called the foundation beam of the head. The pituitary gland sits in a saddle-like indentation exactly in the middle of this bone. To make it easy for the baby to go through the birth canal, the sphenoid is in three parts during labor. Our task is to make sure that these three parts, which go through all kinds of twists and compressions, grow together in a most ideal way so maximum space is available.

### Treatment

Place your thumbs at the temples by the side of the eyes in the little indentations until you feel movement. Let yourself go with the movement in order for the bones to express themselves, and then show them exactly, with your full intention, where their right place is. **Wait until balance arises.**

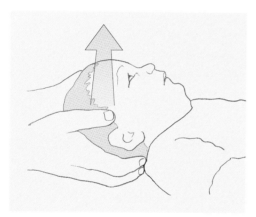

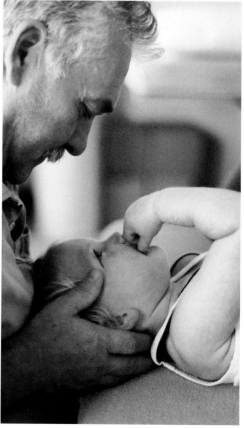

## CHAPTER 7

# Damage Control Is Sometimes Necessary

If the baby is stuck during birth, all help is welcome—we do want to live! There are three methods that save many lives every year: forceps, suction, and cesarean (C-section).

### Forceps

- This tool that looks like it was invented during the Inquisition can be used with the appropriate delicacy by an experienced obstetrician. Compression of the head is secondary to survival. Luckily, we can repair most if not all damage.

The sphenoid, which lies behind the eyes and in between the temples, can become permanently tilted, because it is in three parts at birth and is easily displaced. It can be shifted due to both normal birth compression and forceful extraction.

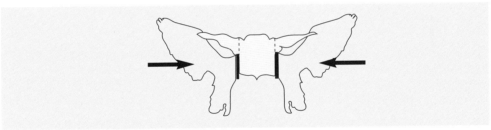

Compressive forces that will arise during birth can become excessive when a forceps is used. The dark lines in the middle show the parts that are still flexible to accommodate the birth compression.

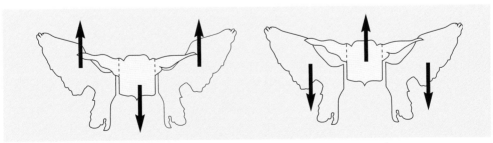

The way the baby chooses to be born and devices like the suction cup can produce all kinds of dragging forces on the three parts of the sphenoid.

### Treatment

Treatments are done mainly by decompression techniques, especially V-spread,* finger in the mouth, CV4, and freeing up of the whole CS system.

## Vacuum Pump (suction apparatus)

- The special structure of the little head with its big fontanel at the top makes it extremely vulnerable when this suction apparatus is used. The nature of the instrument invites the use of force instead of delicacy in the treatment. Luckily our neo-cortex (big brain or cerebrum) hasn't started its final development. Distortions in the ventricles and their relationships with the very fine capillaries will always happen, and this will deregulate the making of and distribution of CS fluid. Little heads that go through this feel as if the suction cup is still on there, that the fluid inside the head is still compressed and that there is a power in there which cannot escape.

### Treatment

Let one hand be on top of the head and find the right spot, while you support the occiput with the other hand. Your attention will be drawn into the ventricles. Let yourself come to rest, so that the fluid can absorb your easiness. Everything will slowly, slowly, slowly regulate itself through this communion, the wordless communication with the life-force.

In the given situation, the baby didn't have any other choice than to submit itself fully to this procedure. Often it seems calm and content. This quiet layer will hide a deeper one, filled with frustration, fear and anger that will, of course, need to be expressed, ideally during the session. The parents and therapist need to understand that the screaming isn't directed at them personally; it is pure frustration created by pain and helplessness, but also a cry for help.

---

* V-spread is used when you want to send a lot of energy to a specific point, so stuck energy or pain can move or dissolve. It is usually done by holding the point or area you want to address in one hand (with V-spread fingers or the cup of your hand), and with the other hand you send energy to that specific spot from the opposite side of the body.

## The Acute Cesarean

- When a little baby gets stuck during labor and the compression forces become too dangerous, a cesarean can be the only option. The belly of the mother will be cut open, and when the little unborn child's body is removed, it experiences a sudden change in pressure. Instead of being compressed, it experiences a sudden decompression, and its little head suddenly expands. To complete the extraction, the little body is being pulled out against its natural birth direction. The sedation given to the mother can also end up in the body of the baby and it may have an experience of being "paralyzed" in the middle of its first life task. Finally the bonding ritual may be postponed, sometimes for a few weeks, because of the necessary medical care for the mother. Of course, the little baby has no other choice than to accept this treatment completely, and again, frustration, fear and anger may be repressed. It is necessary that the mother be made aware of all these physical aspects so she can understand the impact it has on her little one and compensate for it. It is also absolutely necessary to make everybody understand that this intrusion was the best that could be done, given the circumstances.

### Treatment

Going softly/firmly over the whole body of the baby with both hands together, from the top of the head to the tips of the feet, is a good way to awaken the idea of the right direction and the right rhythm. It is grounding. These children haven't finished something, as if they didn't incarnate in their bodies fully. The main goal of the treatment is directed to the completion of the natural birth, where they learn to use gravity as their ally and also get a chance to be really born through an improvised birth canal. Treatment happens mainly in the slowest CS rhythms where the empowerment of the rhythm is the main goal. Here the little body of the baby will learn from the body of the therapist. During the treatment, while the little body is in an unwinding* process, the

---

\* Unwinding is a known term in CS therapy. The therapist supports the body in such a way that it feels weightless. Muscles, organs, and bones that always have to take gravity into account will get a sense of a freedom they don't know and will start making movements that are otherwise impossible or prohibited for them. Unwinding creates an immense sense of freedom and joy in the body.

head will start to get a feel of gravity. The inside of the head as well as the fluid will be begging for gravity. Let yourself come to rest within the very first movements; slow them down for yourself. Often a full-body unwinding will take place, and I will knead all muscle groups and organs, including sacrum and pelvis; sometimes I do a lot of techniques, and sometimes I do very little. Whatever I do will always be followed by treatment of atlas/occiput and head.

### The Planned Cesarean (indications or when)
- Some babies' heads are just too big for the birth canal or there are other complications. The doctor chooses what he/she thinks is the right moment to cut the baby out of the mother. The natural birth compression in the body of the baby will not be activated, and the biological clock of mother and baby can be compromised.

- Fear of pain during labor, the "nip and tuck" culture, or unresolved birth traumas in the mother can cause the mother to ask for a planned cesarean. Sometimes there isn't enough time, willingness or energy to resolve one's own deep fears—after all, it is a rather large parcel heading for a small opening.

- I have heard that some obstetricians will change the natural rhythm of babies so it will fit in with their schedule. Also, cesareans might diminish the possibility of lawsuits. In some countries (according to Chilton Pearce) they really go overboard.

- The birth clock which regulates the natural rhythms and body systems in mother and child will become completely confused. Here also the parents need to know that the little baby has no other choice than to accept this drastic and unnatural way of "labor interruptus." And here too, sometimes the seemingly quiet baby hides a lot of frustration, anger, and fear. Of course during the treatment all these layers need to be addressed and expressed—remember it is not directed personally at the parents or the therapist. It is a release of blocked energy and it is not pleasant.

#### Treatment
This happens by consoling the baby, holding the baby and giving it the opportunity to express itself. This should be done preferably

in the arms of the mother. As mentioned above, softly/firmly going over the whole body from top to bottom with both hands will awaken the original direction and compression of birth. A soft pressure against the feet while simultaneously activating the "whirling" memories in the spine will allow the baby to start up and fulfill its real birth process. In particular, activating its CS rhythm will empower the CS fluid and maximize the baby's energy (sending of energy upwards via the sacrum or the navel).

*My youngest son was in his second year of medical school and was sitting in a coffee shop with a few friends when an over-excited man came running in: his wife was in the car giving birth in the back seat, and he was asking if there was a doctor in the house. There wasn't, but the friends let the man know: "Here is a medical student."*

*My son went to the car and was just in time to bring a nice baby into the world. Everybody thought: "This is a sign from existence—this medical student will become a perfect obstetrician." And so that became his plan, until he heard about the legal aspects. Lawsuits and insurance against lawsuits kill the pleasure that needs to be fundamentally present in a doctor.*

*I also remember my daughter, who absolutely wanted to give birth in her own home. Her little class of prospective mothers was shown, three weeks before she was due, about everything that can go wrong when you give birth at home. Needless to say they all went to the hospital, and on top of that, more than half of them chose a C-section, including her.*

### Next ... what can we do for the mother after a C-section?
Cutting open the belly, the muscles, and the uterus also cuts through a lot of acupuncture meridians, which gives rise to dysfunctions in many organs and in the energy distribution throughout the whole body. These problems can sometimes take years to manifest themselves. It is a true testament to mothers and their happiness that many of them recuperate as fast as they do.

Of course, fathers and therapists can be a tremendous help in these times, and a therapist can teach fathers little tricks that will help the mother.

### Treatments for the Mother

- Start at the base of the nails of the small toes, left and right at the outside; here you touch the bladder meridian (which connects to the kidney meridian). Create balance between left and right. With a little practice you will be able to feel where the meridian is disconnected. Breathe easily—there is nothing you have to do. The energy will do the work for you; you just wait for a feeling of balance.

- Place your fingers on the second small toe; here you find the gall bladder meridian, which will connect with the liver meridian. Again you do nothing, you just wait for balance. If your fingers want to connect with the first two little toes, just let them do what they want.

- Go to the crevice between the big toe and the four others, just on the foot and in between the tendons; here you find the spleen meridian, which is connected to the stomach, and do the same.

- Place your hands under the calves, with one fingertip exactly in the little fold where the two calf muscles separate; you'll notice that the palms of your hands will touch the outside of the legs just above the ankles. The mother will feel a tremendous relaxation in her uterus. Sometimes I start with this one even before I go to the toes.

- Then you do fascia release on the wound, the whole belly, pelvic diaphragm, and wherever you feel it to be necessary.

### The Use of Anesthetics

Sedation, so you won't feel any pain at all, is surely possible in our modern times. You ask, "Why should I feel pain?" That the baby may also get sedated is not usually a consideration. The new body will find the first signals coming from the world it is traveling to a little bit confusing. It is as if you are invited to go on your first-ever field trip, but suddenly your legs and arms won't work. That this can lead to difficulties in dealing with stress seems to me evident. Some specialists attribute drug use in later life to these first signals. I do not only mean the use of illegal drugs, but I wouldn't be surprised if the big pharmaceutical companies are on a par with the nicotine distributors. This is pure deduction on my part; it is common sense and has no scientific or legal basis at all (that I am aware of), so do not sue me!

**Treatment**

This happens by maximizing the flow of the CS fluid. I often involve the thymus. Intention wants to find the "mist" and remove it from the body. Relax fully, find the mist, and find a way out for the mist; then you can fill that newfound clarity with CS fluid and energy.

## CHAPTER 8

# Being Born and Dying...
# One and the Same?

Being born and dying are two almost symmetrical events, with life in between. It's a good thing to connect these two dramas to each other, because each can give insights into the other and they can also supplement each other. The soul needs nine months to consolidate from pure energy into a form where this energy can be contained in matter. Also, to hold onto something, energy is needed. When this life-energy is used up, the body starts losing its grip on the soul, and it will also take nine months for this process to take place in a quiet and complete manner. During this slow process of letting go, deep problems might rise to the surface because, to hide problems, one needs a lot of energy. That's also one of the reasons why the older we get, when our energy potential starts to fade, little by little all kinds of defects show themselves. This process of letting go occurs on another level every day; we call it sleep and it is nothing more than our daily "little death."

Approaching the end of life is the best time to make balance in your life, and to make peace wherever that is possible, until finally the soul is ready to return to the spot from where it had once come. Saying goodbye to the body can be practiced during life, and the same thing is true about being born. The soon-to-be mother can make her own cells *and* also the cells of the child ready for the arrival of a soul in a human form.

If problems are not recognized or released, they will stick to the soul. This soul will feel the need to materialize again and again because these problems can only be resolved here, where you got them. Some souls will even stick to each other and will have to share and solve their karma here on Earth, attracted by their common heavy stickiness.

When we take our client back, closer and closer to the birth, the memory of the place where he or she came from will arise and become deeper. It is the place where your birth-plan—that which you need to do in this life—was formulated. If the client can feel and describe this plan again, it becomes easier to put all not-so-pleasant experiences of this life in their true light. Freeing up some of these obstacles will not always be achieved, because the soul also needs certain hindrances and resistances to work out its karma.

During our training as CS therapists we re-experience our conception, time in the womb, and the whole birth process, so we can explore the problems if any arise. With our clients, if necessary, we similarly take them back to the time when problems first began, which can be as early as conception.

## CHAPTER 9

# Gravity: The Stolen Secret!

In all births gravity helps to give direction to the incarnation. Cells use and trust this wisdom; it gives them the feeling that they are on the right path. It is an enormously defining feeling. Throughout your whole life, you can feel from the gravity at birth that you are on the right path!

The tradition of putting mothers on their back makes the birth process a struggle against nature. The whole animal kingdom uses gravity as the defining force to incarnate. In our birthing rooms the male part of society has interfered a little too much. After preventing the passing on of the birth rites by "wise women" (the Inquisition, enforced by a sexually perverted class, priests), the obstetrical male caste decided that every mother should be on her back, so they could see better what was happening. Babies that go through this unnecessary battle against gravity crave the gravitational force as a natural ally. Children who are treated with the help of gravity in the CS techniques, especially after they were born with a cesarean, can make enormous leaps in their development, both physical and mental.

### Treatment
Begin with stretching the spine. The head will start feeling so heavy, it will look for and follow gravity; it is the only natural inclination and ally in this new environment. With the head down a natural rest starts to descend. Take the time to absorb this restfulness. Whatever unwinding happens, just follow it. Afterwards, do the atlas/occiput and skull techniques.

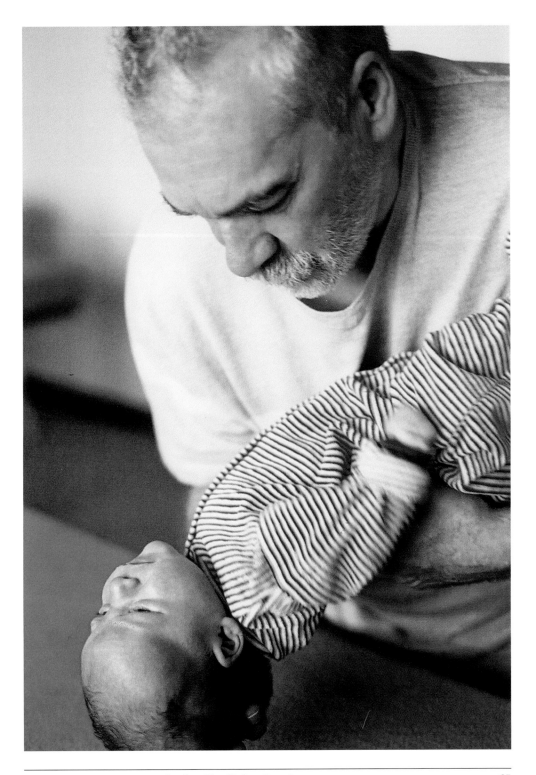

## *SERIES 3* – Reliving Birth to Repair Damages

Because the little girl was shy, I invited the mother and child to be together on the treatment table. Once the mother relaxed it was easy for me to start working with the little girl. Before I knew it, she went into cell memories and her body was looking for the intimacy of the contact with my energy and touch. She came crawling toward me, literally. Without any problem, she let gravity take over and used my hands and body to re-do her full birthing process.

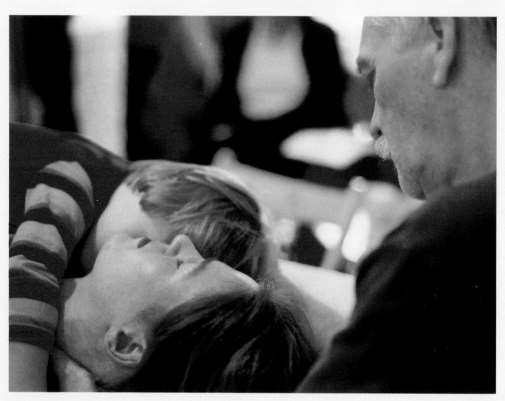

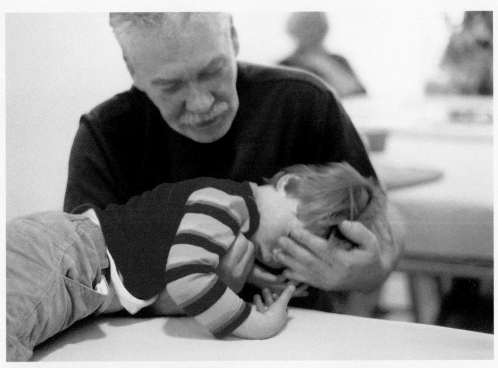

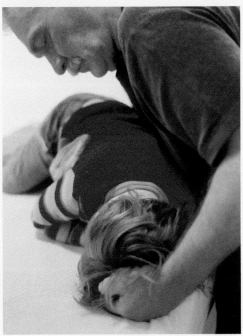

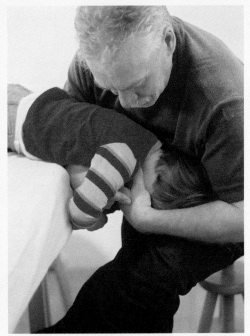

The only thing I had to do was to slow down this experience and give enough pressure with my thighs and knees for her head and body to feel enough counter-pressure to do what needed to be done. While she was born again through my legs, I started to talk very gently, very affirmingly, and asked the mother to sit on the floor so she could catch her own daughter.

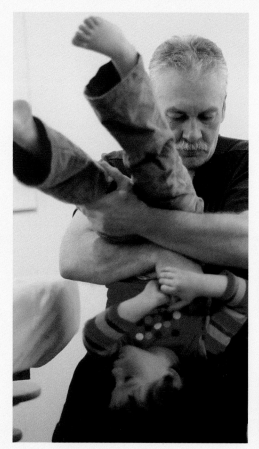 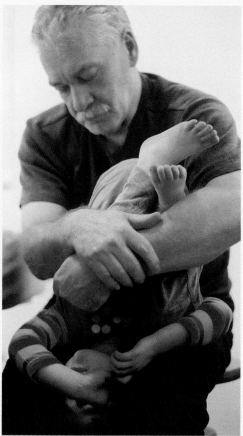

This unwinding is particularly helpful for cesarean-born children, children who haven't fully materialized (spaced-out children), children with learning problems and concentration difficulties. Then, cell memory is a journey in time towards an experience that happened but wasn't fully resolved. Everything will be relived, and it is as if this child (or baby) is completely in a dream.

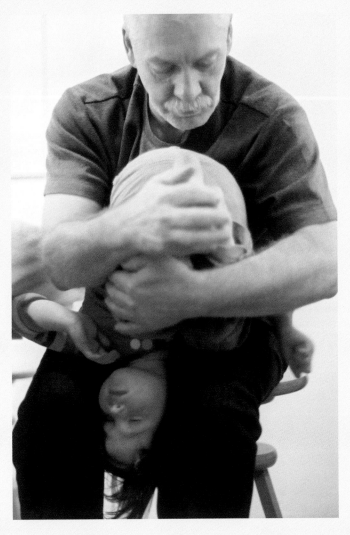

## SERIES 4 – BREECH BIRTH

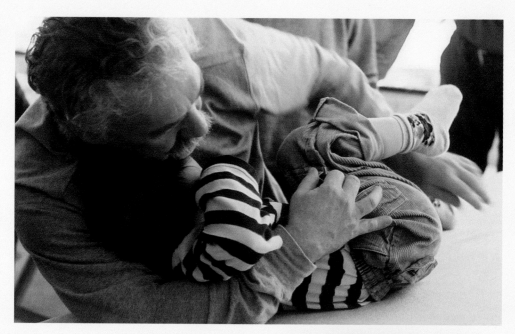

In the picture, gravity is at work and you see the cell memories of the little boy. These kids usually need to make a "statement." I help them to go through their unresolved physical problems first, and often they will be able to do their birth in a head-first way later. Then their grounding gets a new dimension.

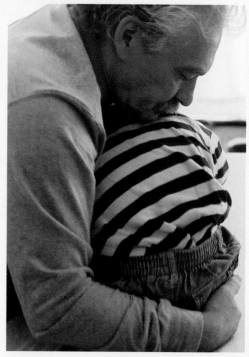

**Craniosacral Therapy for Babies and Small Children**

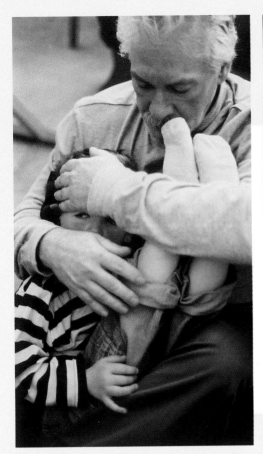

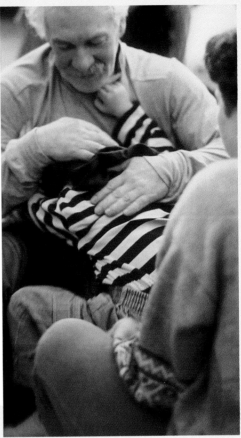

Some kids just choose the hardest way to be born. If the mother knows this in advance, she can ask the unborn child to turn around. Communication between mother and unborn child often happens spontaneously; and if not, we can help the mother to do that in our sessions. There is also a meridian point* that can help the child turn, and if this is done before the beginning of the ninth month, it has a good chance of succeeding.

A good shiatsu practitioner, acupuncturist, or foot reflexologist should be able to help. If bladder 67 is activated (at the outside of the small toe, at the base of the nail), the baby will turn (both sides). It is advisable to do acupressure regularly or heating of the point on the small toes when it is time for the baby to make its final turn.

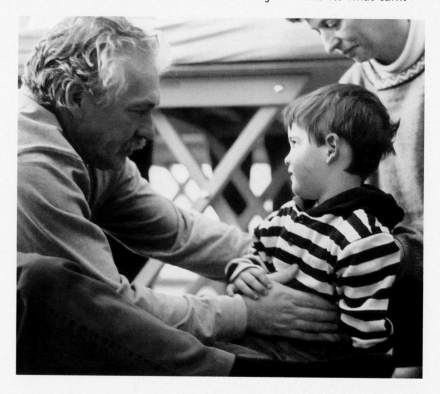

---

* Meridian Points: Open up the whole reproductive area by opening bladder 61 and after that 3 yin-3 yang (spleen-pancreas 6 and gall bladder 39).

## CHAPTER 10

# Your First Impressions
# and Your World

Unconscious feelings that take root during pregnancy and birth:

- Panic is sometimes the first reaction when a woman discovers that she is pregnant, and it can give the baby the feeling that "Is it all my fault?"

- Not enough ease or space in utero and at birth can introduce this world as a dangerous or scary place, especially if, on top of that, you have to fight against gravity.

- The more intimate one is with somebody, the more it's possible to be hurt.

   *This was the case with one of my students, who was frightened to move inside the uterus, because every time she touched the walls of the uterus, she could feel the panic and anguish of her mother. She really froze up when the mother tried to terminate the pregnancy.*

- New situations are always threatening because once you were being squeezed beyond belief and suddenly there was a forceps around your head and you were pulled literally into a new dimension.

- Stress makes you freeze up, like when you wanted to enter the world but suddenly you became paralyzed because of the anesthetics.

- Reaching a goal can equal pain and disaster, because, who knows, maybe another of these suction cups is going to be put on your head and give you pain and confusion all over again.

Our first impressions will underlie our emotional behavior patterns for the rest of our lives.

We have two almond-shaped organs just behind our eyes, the amygdalas, our emotional eyes. They work like radar and track all dangerous and maybe life-threatening emotional energies.* The alarm from the amygdalas activates the release of stress hormones, and if your reaction towards the energies was successful, this response will be saved for further use by our most primitive memory, the hippocampus.

> *If your brother is always pinching you or shows his jealousy in another way, you're going to scream to make your mother come and tell your brother off. If this happens a few times, your system will start recognizing the energy of your brother as threatening and you will release stress hormones whenever he looks like he's going to behave like that, so you start screaming and calling for help from the mother. If your mother is not in the neighborhood, your system will release the same stress hormones if you feel your brother coming close ... even until the present! The hippocampus in its turn also has to give the signal to stop the production of stress hormones when your body is being flooded with them. We learned the full response to a threatening situation, and with every situation of the same kind in the future, we have a ready-made and immediate response at hand, again, making sure our safety is guaranteed.*

The amygdalas and hippocampus reside almost in the middle of our head, and therefore absorb enormous pressure during labor contractions, or can get displaced by use of the suction cup. Experiences like that ensure that these stress-regulators are often taxed to the limit.

### Treatment

The primary response of a baby is to the sound of its mother's heartbeat, the rushing of the blood, and the sounds that organs make. Your voice and its intention, not its words, make the connection with this new life. Then you softly introduce your touch while you make soft easy words and sounds. I never use so-called "baby language" because I am talking to a soul and not to an

---

* You can find a complete explanation in Daniel Goleman's book, *Emotional Intelligence* (London: Bloomsbury Publishing, 1996).

idiot. Hold this commitment and communicate your intention and what you want to do, with your whole body. Let the child know that he/she is welcome and that you want to help.

**This is the moment that I, as a therapist, become love.**

*When I saw my wife talk to one of our fresh new grand-children, I understood really the beginning of the Bible: "In the beginning was the word, and the word became light."*

After unity is restored in this way, if you gain access and acceptance from the baby, it might make eye contact with you.*

- A baby that has just gone through hell will first have to re-experience unity with its mother before it can accept you. **No is no.** A little trick to circumvent this "no" is to treat the mother first. As mentioned before, mothers are so full of caring that they will almost always run ahead of themselves. A treatment will make a huge difference for her, and so the little trick works both ways. The further the mother goes into relaxation, the quieter the baby will become. Then I will extend my attention into treating mother and baby as a unity, and even start touching the baby (even if from a distance) and afterwards also physically.

- Speak slowly and directly to the child. Tell the baby if you need to ask something of the parents and wait (!) until it gives a response before talking to the parents. Give the baby the time to hear you and to understand you—wait for its response! Never forget that babies come from a timeless space and for every question that you ask they have to create brand-new neural circuits.

---

* During research, brains of newborns were connected to a computer via electrodes. Every time the researcher or the mother really looked into the baby's eyes, the instruments showed maximum brain capacity and shut down whenever one looked away. Research also shows that neurons grow when they are stimulated, such as with eye contact, touch, or the making of slow, familiar sounds. We also know how we can prevent or kill the growth of neurons, especially those of the prefrontal cortex, just by giving negative commands, like saying "no" to everything the baby wants to experiment with, or "watch out" whenever a child wants to investigate a new experience.

- Expansion techniques (EV4) are the equivalent of love; you expand the system in order for life energy to fill it up. This is especially valuable with deep traumas.

- Let your fingers show you the way; do nothing until the body uses your energy to steer your hands.

- Your body is the guide for the bones of the baby. Sometimes you have to show them their place; there are no barriers yet, so you can show exactly where every bone can fulfill its life task maximally.

- Life has three basic intentions: power, in order to create space; and space, so that it can recognize itself. The third intention is the return to unity.

## CHAPTER 11

# What is the Ideal Preparation for a Soon-to-be Mother?

The most fundamental thing that you can give to a mother-to-be is to give her back her notochord; in other words, we connect her again deeply with her **mid-line** within the dural tube. During the treatments all her cells, everything, will literally be put in alignment. The power that arises from this very deep space will connect the mother again to her deepest knowing. On top of that, it will become an earned rite which she can fall back on during labor. Accompanying the mother during labor with CS therapy will give mother and child a natural ally. Everybody who is helping will be able to feel this most natural of rhythms; it will tell when to push and when to wait.

### Treatment
- All known CS techniques, but mainly the three compression spots (atlas/occiput, occiput/sphenoid, and L5 S1).

- Giving space to organs that have to give way to the expanding uterus, and especially giving a lot of attention to the respiratory diaphragm.

- All deep tissue and fascia techniques (around the pelvis).

- In an ideal world mother will be treated before and after birth by a CS therapist, or even better, if mother has the time and space to learn basic CS therapy techniques, she can claim back many of the stolen birth rites.

*During our CS courses, we regularly have pregnant women as students. In one of our follow-up trainings around Sutherland's lesions we even had a student who was ready to give birth at any moment. She had contact with her baby the whole time and she felt completely secure. Needless to say, this security arose from regular CS treatments. Exactly a week after the training her baby was born very quietly.*

## CHAPTER 12

# Is There a Task
# for the Father?

After deliverance of the DNA in the head of the sperm, the father doesn't play a role as far as building the baby is concerned. The body of the mother will build the baby cell by cell. After that, the mother will feed the baby with milk that she produces. For me, as a man, this is something that I can only observe in wonderment without feeling the hormonal impact of it all.

We men can provide support, food, and security! In an ideal world, and pregnancy is an ideal world for the mother on a hormonal level, the man will feed the mother in all possible ways and give her the necessary security so she can devote herself fully to building a complete child. Passion, softness, and love will nurture the soul and body of the mother so deeply that the physical formation of this small growing child will become the most natural thing on Earth. In a world where our priorities are not necessarily also natural priorities, this is the only possible solution. The fun thing is, that if the father takes this role upon himself, there will awaken a deep hormonal feeling of protection in him; the "lord of the manor" (the father) will be born and fulfill and fill both their lives. Evolution is guaranteed and possibilities are again limitless.

It is clear that fighting between mother and father will always break down what is hormonally planned. This means confusion and stagnation on all levels of the unit for mother, father, and child. It is our observation that some parents will stubbornly avoid therapeutic intervention so they can, unconsciously, pass on their neuroses to their children.

In our SETR treatments (somato emotional trauma release) we can investigate with the soon-to-be mother or father what it is that sabotages or hinders a pregnancy. We are able to look objectively at their traumas and difficulties and respond to them like: "Is this response valid at this moment? Can we change this response, and if not, what is necessary to change it?" This way we can look at the client's problem and find a way to release what got stuck long ago. With SETR during the treatment, we talk with the client about cell memories. Together with the client, these unsolved memories are spoken about, looked at, and resolved.

## CHAPTER 13

# What Can Hinder
# or Make a Pregnancy Difficult?

Not every woman who wishes it is ready to become pregnant.

> *Lieve wanted to become pregnant but was unable to. During treatments we soon found out that things had happened in early childhood that had convinced her heart-protector\* that intimacy was threatening to the integrity of her heart. To avoid this danger the heart-protector had put a firm harness around her heart that extended around her physical body. Nothing was allowed in and almost nothing could escape.*

In our early childhood, when our heart is really vulnerable, a heart-protector will guarantee the integrity of the heart. However, we never thank the heart-protector; we never say, "Thank you. I have survived and I can stand on my own feet now. I am a grown-up, I make my own decisions, and I am not dependent anymore on the people who have raised me. So, please, lighten up a little, my heart needs to make connections and in order to do that I need to feel emotion and I need to show emotion!"

If you don't communicate, this heart-protector will remain like a harness; and it will become impossible for you to show love or to receive love freely. We can show your heart-protector that other helpers have grown in your body (like your voice, the power in your eyes) and that you are grown up and able to protect the heart fully. The heart-protector will never stop protecting the integrity of the heart: don't forget what is at stake. Once your protector understands and loosens up, your heart can finally relax; on top of that you stay safe, because the heart-protector has new helpers and also has regained flexibility to open or close whenever or whatever is needed.

---

\* The heart-protector (pericardium) is the physical membrane made from tough fascia that sits around the heart and has its own meridian. It sits in the middle of the chest on top of the respiratory diaphragm. It starts its task as an emotion-protector for the heart very early in utero.

*To go back to our example of Lieve: this woman of thirty years was still being protected by a heart-protector that learned its task when she was three. Afterwards, no correction had been made. During the session the pericardium became convinced that its owner had developed new means of protecting her integrity, especially her voice. The originator of the malice had passed away years before, and the protector was willing to cooperate so that she could stand in life as the grown-up that she was. Finally the heart-protector became convinced that for an adult heart to be able to survive and fulfill its life task, adult nurturing like love and intimacy was an absolute necessity. She became so spacious that the heart and uterus were allowed to accept whatever was needed for them to fulfill their life task (in a screened way, i.e., opening her protector but with awareness). A beautiful little girl was conceived soon after with the help and support of a heart-protector that became grown up and conscious.*

### Considerations and Recommendations

- Some organs will resist a pregnancy at all costs. They will need to be convinced that their owner has become an adult.

- To work on yourself means resolving dysfunctional sympathetic and parasympathetic patterns in particular, and also regulating the reticular alarm system (RAS).

- Unrecognized and therefore unresolved birth traumas of the mother will probably be passed on to the baby.

- I prefer to tell all organs or parts of the brain about the pregnancy. Initiating this dialogue between the client and her own body shows that in every organ and even in every cell, consciousness is present. If this is recognized and practiced, a whole new relationship between the client and her body arises. The body then becomes a conscious partner, guardian, and helper with a completely different view of reality.

- A mother who works to solve her own problems will always invite souls who fit in with that level of consciousness.

- After an abortion there is often so much guilt and sadness because it was very difficult to say farewell to the soul that wasn't welcome. If this is the case, saying farewell will still need to happen. The dialogue between the mother and the soul that may still be hanging around is often very emotional. Fear of this burden, and unforgiving and unevolved views of religion and society, play a big part in the inability of the mother to let it go. Compare this situation with a car that doesn't work but is still in your garage. There is no space for a new one!

- If a pregnancy is not wanted, this can be explained to the unborn soul and you can ask the soul to leave the body of the fetus before the pregnancy is terminated. All guilt needs to be addressed and discussed among all the partners (the soul, the mother, and all the organs that are involved).

- When labor is getting near, I tell the body of the mother and also the body of the baby what they can expect at the birth time. I ask the pituitary and the spinal cord to produce enough oxytocin and endorphins.

- We do everything we can to motivate the mother to breast-feed her baby, and we can also ask the pituitary gland to produce enough prolactin to activate the milk production.

- A skilled practitioner can communicate with the CS rhythm of the unborn baby, and eventually can ask advice about anything that can help.

- Eventually you can also ask the baby in utero when it wants to be born, on which day, or if need be, you can tell the baby it is going to have a cesarean birth.

CHAPTER 14

# Where, Dear Soul,
# Do You Come From?

If you want to say something that makes sense about the place you came from, it would be that it is a place of unity (oneness). If you want to look at this oneness you need to use a trick; you have to get out of it. It is literally a trick because, if you are "one," how can you look at it? It is the game that we play: to forget our unity so we can find it back. It is a game with many rules because you need a body; in the body you need DNA and emotions; and before you know it, you need eternity just to get to know the toy that you are using.

At a certain moment the soul is ready to separate from the whole and become a body in this world. After a few journeys you don't want to be a fish anymore, you want to be a fisherman. So you formulate an itinerary or life-task and the only thing you are waiting patiently for is the exact circumstances as you want them to be, so they will fit your itinerary. Then, with your itinerary locked in your DNA, the day arises that you can't hold back anymore, because two people are making love and by doing so, they send out a signal into the cosmos—one return ticket to Earth! The invitation that has been sent can read as follows: "We, both of us, want a sweet and lovely child, but it needs to be a boy, because we need a boy to continue our family name or business." Of course, if you read this invitation and your plan is to experience life as a girl, how can you keep on loving yourself? Here is your chance. Most invitations that are sent read, "We are horny, we don't have condoms, we confuse physical attraction with love, so we will be really shocked if somebody accepts this invitation, because we, ourselves, don't even know that this is an invitation" or "I have just been raped; is there somebody out there who is willing to be my child?" Just like in a good store for birth cards, on the cosmic level you can find any invitation you can imagine. There is a moment when the invitation is being sent out.

Of course there are always a lot of souls ready to start a "working vacation." This is the moment when formless energy will be caught again in an energy field and will incarnate into matter. Here is the beginning of form, the limitation of space and so the beginning of time. All conditions are now fulfilled to proceed further with investigating what our consciousness needs to find here. The invitation for the soul will always come at the right moment, because time is a phenomenon that only exists here. It is remarkable to see that the soul never chooses your next-door neighbor, or those people from across the street with the Mercedes, but always ends up with those you now call Mommy and Daddy.

Most of the time the strongest and fastest sperm will get the chance to penetrate the egg. But in the best of worlds, conception will be the result of a culmination of love, filled with ecstasy in which time and space are replaced by total unity. Under this circumstance the seed with the exact energetic key, that carries the exact spiritual ecstasy in itself, will be allowed. One seed out of millions, the one with the right kundalini, will start a controlled nuclear reaction that will last its whole life.

An important part of our CS treatments is to bring the client back in the past to the moment before conception. There they can clearly reconnect with their itinerary, and it is our task to help the client see this in all its simplicity. This is mostly a tremendous support when clients cannot accept all that they have gone through because of their parents, schools, or relationships. Their life-plan will then be seen in the perspective of their true origin, and letting go of excessive baggage will become easier.

## *SERIES 5 -* A Beautiful Visitor

This series gives a clear picture of a full session. This session stands out as one of those that happened completely in "no-time." It was a treatment in which there was no thinking at all. The complete session happened in the slowest of all CS rhythms where time and thinking are absent. It is a world of space and energy. I make a connection between her navel and the fourth ventricle. They are the spots that my hands were attracted to, being the place where for nine months the baby was connected with her mother's energy. You can say that she asked me in via the front door.

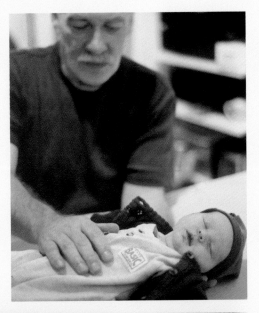

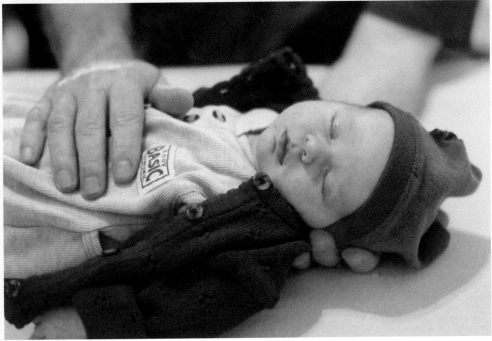

While my right hand moves slowly higher, I listen with my left hand.

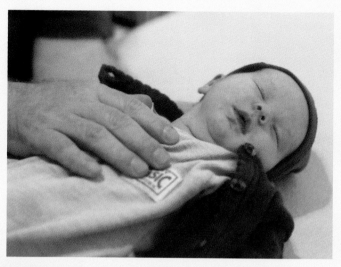

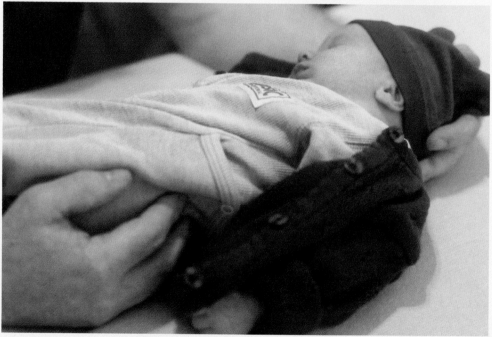

I find a little twist in the spine and follow this as slowly as possible, while I give space with my intention, until everything falls into place.

I am listening to the atlas and occiput with the intention of spreading them out.

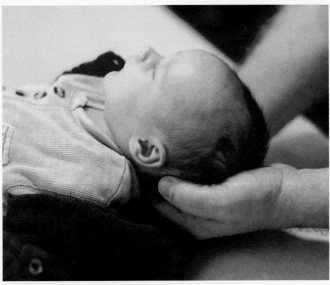

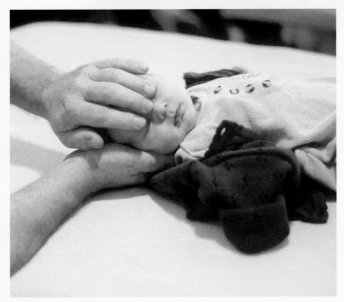

Spreading the condyles with the right hand, the left hand sends energy downwards.

Via the left hand, energy is being sent to the jugular foramen* and after that to the slight compression that I find around the foramen magnum.†

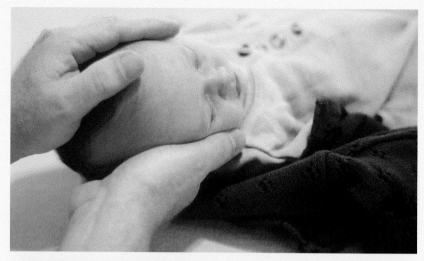

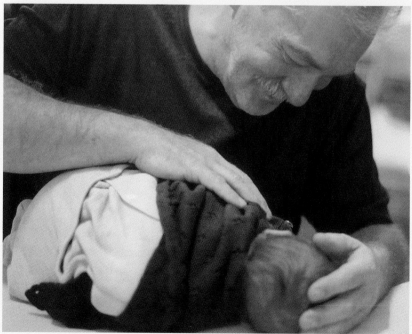

---

* The jugular foramen is a gap between the occiput and the temporal bone deep behind the ears.

† The foramen magnum is the big hole in the occiput where the spinal cord enters the skull.

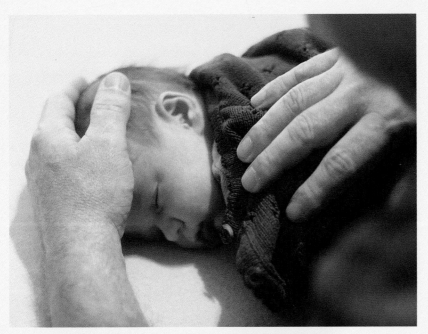

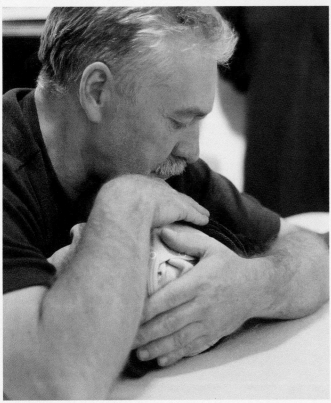

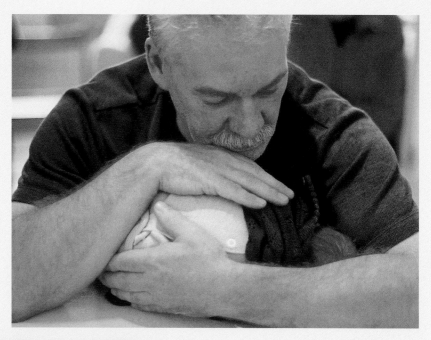

Safety, coziness, and intimacy are words born out of unity.

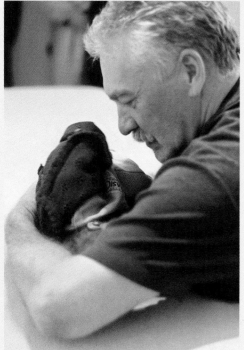

A final check of the spine.

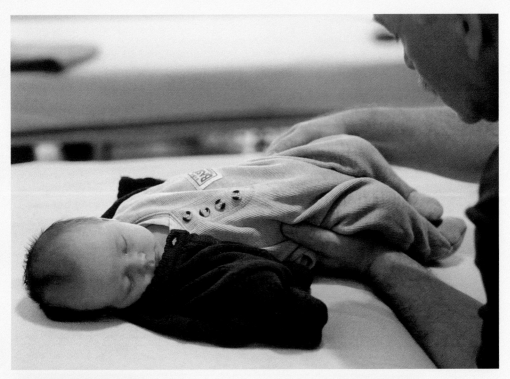

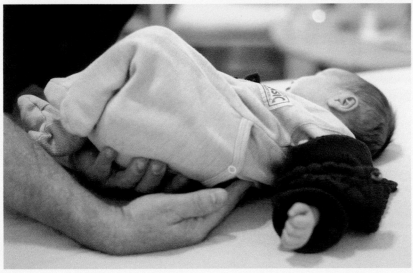

Everything feels fine, have a good life, sweet girl!

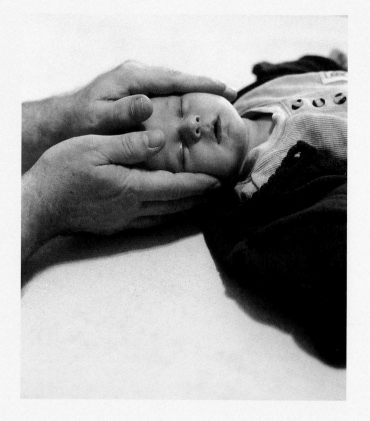

## CHAPTER 15

# Things That You Can
# and Want to Control

- Find a baby-friendly environment or a baby-friendly hospital for the birth; this is an environment where the new baby will be expected as a conscious human being (and not as a number that absolutely shouldn't be born during the weekend).

- "Baby-friendly" also means that baby and mother should get the time to construct their hormonal bonding (unwashed contact on the belly, breastfeeding, no strong light or noise and so on).

- Inoculations, eye drops, and automatic circumcision are not an ideal way to welcome the baby and to allow it the trust that it carries within itself. Inform yourself about inoculations—the link with autism is scary!

- A father who participates is ideal; nowadays there are many courses where both parents learn breathing techniques and how they can support each other during labor.

- Avoid, if possible, all forms of sedation, but if it happens, make sure the mother doesn't end up feeling guilty.

- If a C-section is needed, make sure that all the organs and also the baby know what is coming.

- I know of no cases of sudden infant death syndrome (SIDS) of babies who have had CS treatments.

- Be careful where you are born; where you give birth.

*"Just as the painful ordeal of childbirth finally ended and N.V. (the mother) waited for the nurse to lay her squalling newborn on her chest, the maternity hospital's ritual of extortion began. Before she even glimpsed her baby, she said, a nurse whisked the infant away, and an attendant demanded a bribe. If you want to see your child, families are told, the price is 12 Rupees for a boy and 7 Rupees for a girl. The practice is common here in the city, surveys confirm."*

Bangalore, India
*International Herald Tribune,*
August 30, 2005

• Enjoy your child.

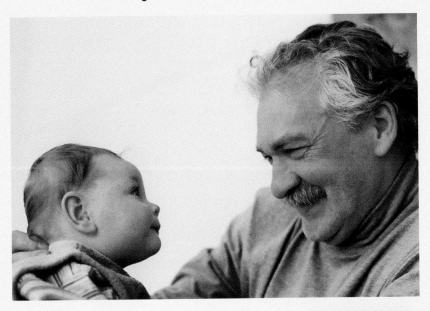

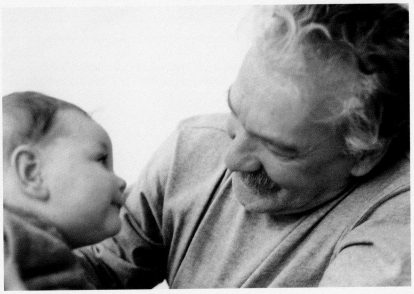

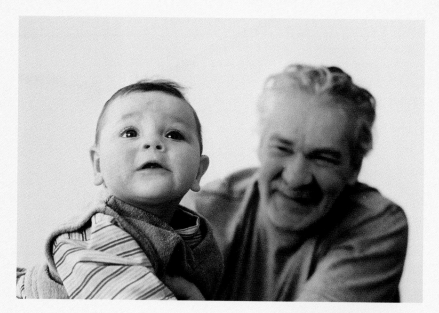

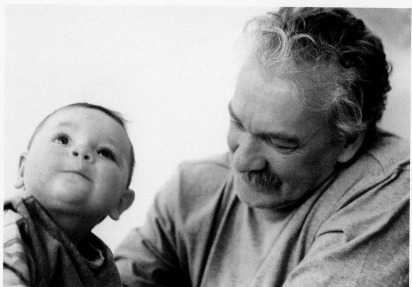

Craniosacral Therapy for Babies and Small Children

# Bibliography

These are books that I read with a lot of pleasure and from which I gathered some information:

Blandine Calais-Germain, *The Female Pelvis*. Seattle, WA: Eastland Press, 2003.

Justine Dobson, *Baby Beautiful*. Carson City, NV: Heirs Press, 1994.

Daniel Goleman, *Emotional Intelligence*. London, England: Bloomsbury Publishing Plc., 1996.

Joseph Chilton Pearce, *The Biology of Transcendence*. Rochester, VT: Park Street Press, 2002.

Nicette Sergueef, *Die Kraniosakrale Osteopathie bei Kindern*. Kotzting/Bayerischer Wald, Germany: Verlag für Osteopathie Dr. Erich Wühr, 1995.

Franklyn Sills, *Craniosacral Biodynamics 2*. Berkeley, CA: North Atlantic Books, 2004.

John Upledger, *A Brain is Born*. Berkeley, CA: North Atlantic Books, 1996.

# About the Authors

Etienne Peirsman (MS Biology) worked as a high school biology and physical education teacher in Antwerp, Belgium, for many years. At a certain point he made a life change and went to India for three years, where he studied meditation, Rebalancing, and CranioSacral therapy. He studied and continues to study with Dr. John Upledger and has been a practicing CranioSacral therapist and teacher for more

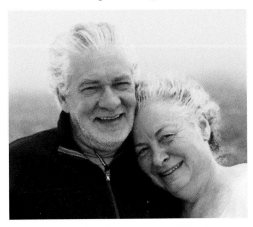

than fifteen years. His unique teaching method brings meditation into the sensitivities of both his clients and students. He lives with his wife in Antwerp, Belgium, and the U.S.

Neeto Peirsman (BA Psychology) worked as a psychiatric assistant in the Fairmount Children's Unit of the Upstate Medical Center in Syracuse, New York, a unit created as a residence for blind children. In 1977 she went to live and work in India for thirteen years, in search of herself. Eventually Etienne also found her and they continue to work as a team in the Cranio field. Presently she works as a private consultant to new mothers.

For more information about Etienne and Neeto's work, please visit www.craniobabies.com.